D1525444

MEDICAL DEVICE ACCIDENTS

With Illustrative Cases

MEDICAL DEVICE ACCIDENTS

With Illustrative Cases

Leslie A. Geddes

CRC Press

Boca Raton   Boston   London   New York   Washington, D.C.

Library of Congress Cataloging-in-Publication Data

Geddes, L. A. (Leslie Alexander), 1921–
    Medical device accidents : with illustrative cases / by Leslie A.
Geddes.
        p. cm.
    Includes bibliographical references and index.
    ISBN 0-8493-9236-5 (alk. paper)
    1. Medical instruments and apparatus--Accidents. I. Title.
    [DNLM: 1. Equipment Failure. 2. Wounds and Injuries--etiology.
    3. Equipment Design. 4. Accident Prevention. WB 26 G295m 1998]
    R856.6.G43   1998
    617.1--dc21
    DNLM/DLC
    for Library of Congress   97-44271
                                                          CIP

No claim to original U.S. Government works
International Standard Book Number 0-8493-9236-5
Library of Congress Card Number 97-44271
Printed in the United States of America 1 2 3 4 5 6 7 8 9 0
Printed on acid-free paper

Contents

Preface

This book is written for all who are concerned with medical device accidents, notably, attorneys, expert witnesses, clinical engineers, nurses, physicians, and manufacturers. Designers of new medical devices will find useful information on how to avoid product misuse or a design defect. The materials presented in the various chapters were drawn from the author's experience preparing and testifying as an expert witness and from teaching biomedical engineers, medical students, and physicians during the last five decades.

The general plan of each chapter is similar. First, the basic principles of a device or a procedure are presented. Then accidents caused by malfunction or misuse of a device are presented. The cause of the accident is identified and explained insofar as possible.

The first chapter deals with product liability and medical technology, in general, and defines product defect, misuse, negligence, and design defect. In addition, statutory medical device reporting and incident reporting are explained. The consequence of two or more technologies being applied to a patient simultaneously, resulting in an accident and injury, is explained.

With the ever-increasing use of electronic controls (analog and digital) in medical devices, their susceptibility to electromagnetic energy is becoming a serious problem. With the rapid growth of the use of high-frequency energy in devices such as cellular telephones, pagers, emergency communications equipment, remote controllers, etc., the amount of electromagnetic interference (EMI) in the environment is increasing at a very rapid rate and medical device malfunction due to EMI is on the increase. Chapter 2 deals with EMI as the cause of malfunction of a variety of medical devices. Such malfunctions have led to serious accidents and deaths. The EMI chapter lists the frequencies used in communications equipment, including AM and FM radio, TV, etc. This chapter describes the malfunction of such devices as apnea monitors, ECG and EEG instruments, ventilators, drug-infusion pumps, pacemakers, automatic implanted defibrillators, and other devices such as motor-driven vehicles. The chapter closes with information on how electrostatic discharge (ESD) can cause medical device malfunction.

The use of high-frequency electric current to cut and coagulate tissue entered surgery in the late 1920s and revolutionized it. Despite the continued improvements in equipment and techniques, electrosurgical accidents are still quite common, ranging from skin burns to bowel-gas explosions and circumcision accidents. The various surgical techniques are described and explanations for the various accidents are presented in Chapter 3.

General anesthesia entered medicine at the middle of the last century with ether (a flammable gas) as the anesthetic agent. Nonflammable gases replaced ether and the anesthetic machine evolved, and to it were added many monitors and alarms.

However, despite all of these improvements anesthetic accidents occur with disturbing frequency. Valves malfunction, the anesthetic circuit develops leaks, and carbon dioxide absorbers become exhausted. Fires occur when oxygen comes in contact with flammable materials that are ignited by a spark from an electrosurgical unit. Such mishaps are described in Chapter 4.

The various mishaps that can occur with intravascular catheters are described in Chapter 5. Despite good manufacturing and good implantation techniques, catheters break and the broken tip migrates, often causing serious injury. In addition, the fluids in catheters can conduct electrical current that can do harm. The forcible injection of contrast medium into the heart can produce an ectopic beat leading to arrhythmias. Many examples of such mishaps are provided.

Direct-current injuries, although infrequent, occur due to device malfunction, misuse, or design defect. Typical injuries due to direct-current are described in Chapter 6.

Transcutaneous Electrical Nerve Stimulation (TENS) is becoming increasingly popular to reduce pain. The technique employs short-duration pulses of current applied to skin-surface electrodes. There is the possibility of such current interfering with implanted electronic devices; this subject is discussed in Chapter 7.

Tissues can be injured thermally, electrically, mechanically, and chemically. The focus of Chapter 8 is pressure and chemical injury, including allergic responses; the other types of injury are discussed in other chapters. Immobility for a period in excess of 2 h invites pressure sores; the nature and the sites of such lesions are discussed in this chapter. The two types of chemical injury, namely, direct-chemical and allergic, are presented. Among the chemicals that produce injury are skin and instrument disinfectants and sterilants. The principle underlying an allergic response and the patch test are explained. Numerous examples of chemical injury and allergic response are given in this chapter.

The last chapter provides hints, tips, and observations derived from the author's experience as an expert witness during trial preparation, deposition, and in the courtroom, which is not the most relaxing environment for a technical expert. However, by knowing the rules and the games that attorneys play, the courtroom can be a place where the expert can play his/her cards to win the game.

I hereby acknowledge the generous assistance given to me by Mark Bruley of the Emergency Care Research Institute (ECRI). He provided many useful reprints and references so that original sources could be found. To Barbara Tincher, my secretary for many years, and to Connie Boss, who joined me recently, I owe a great debt of gratitude for transcribing almost illegible lecture notes that became this book. Both made me feel that the hassle of writing this book was worthwhile. Robert Stern of CRC Press has been the one who kept the project moving and I acknowledge all of his assistance. Finally, the useful suggestions provided by the reviewers of this book are acknowledged; they are R. K. Wright, MD, J D; L. Gyrmek, MD, PhD; and J. Dyro, PhD.

1 Product Liability and Medical Technology

CONTENTS

INTRODUCTION

The law imposes burdens not only on the medical professional who uses technology, but also on the manufacturer, seller, installer, and repairer of technological equipment to insure patient safety. A patient has the right not to be harmed as a result of the use of a medical device, which can be defined as something created to produce a benefit to the patient; it is operated by trained personnel and must not be adversely affected by its working environment.

According to Enghagen (1992), product-liability lawsuits generate more million-dollar-plus judgments than any other class of personal injury, except medical malpractice cases. Therefore, when medical device product liability is associated with medical practice, the stakes can be high and medical device incidents become very serious business. The law imposes burdens to ensure patient safety.

MEDICAL DEVICE EVOLUTION

Since the late 1600s, a variety of electrical (and magnetic) devices were claimed to have a therapeutic effect and were applied widely. The electrostatic machine was used to charge the Leyden jar (capacitor) in 1745, which was then discharged into the body. The discharge was supposed to cure paralysis, diseases of the internal organs, impotence, infertility, psychoses, and a variety of other ailments. Static-electric therapy was succeeded by galvanotherapy, which used direct current, which appeared in the early 1800s. This current was also believed to cure a variety of ailments. Then followed faradic therapy, which employed single or a train of induction-coil shocks to cure illnesses. Then, at the turn of the 20th century, high-frequency current was used to heat body segments to increase blood flow. So popular were these electrical devices that two medical textbooks on their use were published: the first was entitled *A Treatise on Medical Electricity,* authored by J. Althaus and published in Philadelphia in 1873; the second was entitled *On the Medical and Surgical Uses of Electricity,* authored by C. M. Beard and A. D. Rockwell, the 8th edition being published in New York in 1891. Geddes (1984) reviewed the history of these electrotherapeutic techniques.

In this, the Golden Era of Medical Electricity, anecdotal reports were all that was needed to show efficacy and safety. During this time the attitude of the law was "Caveat Emptor" (let the buyer beware). Accidents and failed therapeutic claims resulted in the Pure Food and Drug Act of 1918 in federal regulatory law. In common law, a number of court decisions began to recognize the right to recover monetary damages for injuries caused by products at this time.

By 1938 in the U.S., it became recognized by the lawmakers that the public needed protection against unscrupulous vendors of a variety of medical products. The main concern at that time related to labeling, that is, claims made for the product and the need to remove fraudulent items from the market. In 1938, the Food and Drug Administration (FDA) was given the authority for seizure, injunction, or criminal prosecution with respect to adulterated or misbranded devices. Although numerous cases were tried and many products were removed from the market, the postwar medical instrumentation boom created new jurisdictional problems. After the mid-1940s an enormous variety of medical devices became available to physicians and a large number of these made no claims regarding safety and efficacy. It is important to note that many of these devices played lifesaving roles in the hands of competent physicians. However, many devices had technological flaws. For example, the Federal Register of March 9, 1976 noted that "a committee chaired by Dr. Theodore Cooper, then Director of the National Heart Institute, issued a report indicating that in the 10 years prior to 1969, medical devices caused 10,000 serious injuries and over 750 deaths." An intrauterine device marketed in the early 1970s was linked to 16 deaths and 25 miscarriages. Significant defects in cardiac pacemakers had resulted in 34 voluntary recalls, involving 23,000 units.

Taking note of these facts, the lawmakers passed the Medical Device Legislation Amendments Bill of 1976 (HR-11124, Federal Register, March 9, 1976), which was signed into law. The bill amended the federal Food, Drug, and Cosmetic Act to give it jurisdiction over the safety and effectiveness of medical devices intended for human use in the U.S.

A special feature of this bill allows the FDA to exempt a device from the requirements of the bill if the device is intended solely for investigational use and if the proponent of the device submits a plan demonstrating that the testing of the device will be supervised by an institutional review committee, ensures appropriate patient consent, and maintains certain records and reports. The protocol must be scientifically sound and the benefits and knowledge to be gained must outweigh the risks to the patient. This provision thereby provides a means for the creation of new medical devices.

MEDICAL TECHNOLOGY

Medical technology is advancing at an ever-accelerating rate. New devices and the procedures that they permit are improving the quality of life and prolonging it. Associated with use of the new devices is an increasing number of product-liability lawsuits, often not related to a product defect, but because of new technologies coming together, the patient being the interface. Situations are arising in which two or more medical devices are used on a patient and injury or death results, despite the fact that when tested, the individual devices function normally. In other words, accidents can result from the use of multiple devices connected to a patient.

Despite the fact that there are now rigidly enforced standards for all medical devices, accidents do occur due to medical device malfunction. According to Silberberg (1995) the FDA receives over 95,000 medical device problem reports per year. Many of the incidents that generated the reports involved injury or death to a patient. An increasing number of these incidents involve environmental electromagnetic interference (EMI), which causes medical devices to malfunction. Silberberg (1995) stated:

> Between 1979 and 1995, the Center for Devices and Radiological Health (CDRH) of the U.S. Food and Drug Administration (U.S. FDA) has received over one hundred reports alleging that electromagnetic interference (EMI) resulted in malfunction of electronic medical devices.

Although medical-device accidents are covered in detail elsewhere in this book, a few examples will illustrate the foregoing.

About 100,000 cardiac pacemakers are implanted annually. These sophisticated stimulators can be interrogated and programmed by an external device that uses a radiofrequency link. Patients with pacemakers often undergo surgical procedures that employ electrosurgery, which uses radiofrequency current. There have been cases in which pacemakers caused serious arrhythmias and were reprogrammed, inhibited, and even destroyed when the electrosurgical unit was employed. While the two technologies are safe and effective when used alone, their combination has resulted in injury.

Cellular telephones are used by more and more people, some of whom may be hospitalized and connected to a drug-infusion pump, a dialysis machine, or a monitor. Because the patient has little to do, he/she can pass the time using the cellular phone to talk to friends or family. There have been many instances of malfunction of drug-infusion pumps and patient monitors associated with the use of a cellular telephone. To solve this problem, many hospitals have banned the use of cellular telephones in some areas. Again each technology is safe and effective when operated alone, but malfunction occurred when the technologies came together.

Electrical impedance-based respiration monitors pass a low-intensity, high-frequency current through the chest and detect the increase and decrease in impedance with inspiration and expiration. Such devices alarm when the respiratory rate exceeds a preset low and high breathing rate. However, some such apnea monitors are sensitive to environmental electromagnetic interference (EMI) and fail to alarm. Although safe and effective in low EMI environments, they are not in a high EMI environment.

An example of a potentially serious ECG misdiagnosis was reported by Capuano et al. (1993), who described an ominous arrhythmia in the ECG of a patient whose urine output was being measured by an electronic device. When the urine monitor was turned off, the "cardiac arrhythmia" disappeared. The "arrhythmia", resembling ventricular tachycardia, was traced to beat frequencies between the isolation methods used in the ECG and the urine monitor. Again, each monitor functioned normally, but the combination, when connected to the patient, produced what mimicked a dangerous cardiac arrhythmia. There is therefore an urgent need to "harden" medical devices so that they will be immune from interference sources that are likely to be encountered in the vicinity of a patient. The term "harden" is well known to the military and describes their efforts to make electronic military devices immune from EMI generated by the enemy as well as from environmental sources. Such hardening techniques are well known to civilian engineers and may become a requirement as more EMI-generating equipment appears.

A most important factor in reducing medical device-related accidents is the education of those who use them. The delivery of appropriate education has not kept pace with the appearance of new medical devices that are susceptible to environmental factors. It should not be concluded that education has been totally neglected; it has not. Manufacturers present in-service courses that relate to the proper use of their equipment; but they now need to educate about the hazards of combinations of technologies as well as environmental factors.

It has been said that the best way to keep information away from users of medical devices is to place it in the instruction manual. It has been a constant surprise to the author to discover, during litigation, that many users of medical devices have never read the instruction manual. It should be a rule that before operating a medical device, the operator should be required to prove that he/she has read the manual, no matter how good the in-service training may be or no matter how obvious it is to use the device.

Too little attention is paid to misuse and the effect that environmental hazards may have on a given medical device. Attention to these two factors may well reduce the number of lawsuits; it will certainly reduce the number of defendants per lawsuit.

PRODUCT LIABILITY

Product liability is the term used to describe the litigation in which a complaining party (*the plaintiff*) alleges that a product caused personal injury, property damage, or both and wants to be compensated for the loss by one or more parties (*the defendants*), who may be, and usually include, the manufacturer, contractor, assembler, distributor, vendor, or practitioner who used the product. Product liability is under the purview of civil law and to prevail requires that proof be established by a preponderance of the evidence. The dictionary definition of preponderant is "superior in weight, number, or power". A loose definition of adequate proof would be "more likely than not". This is a lesser requirement than is needed in criminal law where the plaintiff (state, people, or government) must prove its case beyond a reasonable doubt.

Product liability extends into three areas: (1) manufacturing, (2) design, and (3) misrepresentation. To prevail it must be proven that (1) the defect existed when the product left control of the manufacturer or vendor, (2) the provider knew (or should have known) existence of the defect, (3) there were feasible alternatives that would have eliminated the risk, and (4) the product caused the injuries or damages complained of. In essence, by selling a product, a manufacturer accepts an obligation to the consumer.

The following surround the issues pertaining to a product defect: misuse, design defect, FDA Medical Device Reports, and the Incident Report.

PRODUCT DEFECT

Despite a manufacturer's rigorous inspection and testing to assure efficacy and product safety, accidents still occur associated with the proper and improper use of a product. Often it is not obvious how the product failed and caused the harm. The following paragraphs will outline the factors that relate to a product failure.

A product is defective when it fails to meet the provider's own specifications and applicable industrial and/or governmental standards. However, meeting the requirements of such standards is not enough; it must be shown that the product is safe for any reasonable and foreseeable use. For a product to be classified as defective, it is necessary to prove that the defect was present when the product left the manufacturer's premises. Because a product may pass through one or more vendors, it may be difficult to prove when the defect was induced. It is for this reason that the vendor and the manufacturer are often named as codefendants in a lawsuit.

Inspection and maintenance records are very useful in showing that a product was or was not defective. Manufacturers' instruction manuals often specify the type and frequency of these activities. However, if the maintenance is performed by unauthorized personnel, the manufacturer's warranty becomes void and the manufacturer cannot be held responsible for any harm done by a defective product.

The instruction manual identifies the features, operation, and proper use of a product. The manual often identifies risks and hazards and may cite warnings associated with use of the product; this information is often valuable in explaining the reason for an accident.

Some medical devices are leased and it is the responsibility of the lessor to provide a properly functioning and safe product. Therefore, the lessor's inspection, testing, and maintenance records and proof of adherence to the manufacturer's specifications are important. Such information can be useful in explaining the cause of an accident.

All products have a finite life and despite proper inspection, testing, and maintenance, a product can fail due to a component failure. In such a case it may be difficult to establish culpability. However, maintenance records may show that a particular component failed frequently. In many cases, the FDA Medical Device Reports (see below) should be consulted to discover if the same event has been reported by other users of the same product. If so, then the issue of a design defect arises and calls into question the appropriateness of the selection of the component that failed.

An important aspect of a product defect is identifying the consequence of the defect. In other words, it is essential to show that the presence of the defect caused or contributed to the harm. It should be pointed out that in some cases harm was done that was unrelated to a product defect. One should be alert to the practice of blaming a device when improper use or negligence may have occurred. As will be shown in several chapters, harm can result when two properly functioning devices are used on a patient.

MISUSE

When harm results from the misuse of a product, it is assumed that the product was without a manufacturing or design defect. Therefore, the issue becomes one of user behavior. The Supreme Court held that foreseeability is significant in product-liability cases when the product is what it is intended and known to be, but injury is suffered because the product is misused. A product is not misused merely because the manufacturer intended that it be used in a different manner; the manufacturer must show that the use which caused the injury was not reasonably foreseeable. Therefore, the manufacturer is responsible for designing a product with reasonable misuse in mind, as well as communicating the features of the product to the user. It is in this area that the instruction manual can play an important role.

There are two elements in misuse: (1) contributory negligence and (2) assumption of risk. In the former case, the test of reasonableness applies. In other words, did the user act as a reasonable person in the same or similar circumstances? In the latter case, the assumption of risk is evaluated on the basis of what the user knew just before the incident. In assessing the assumption of risk, there are three elements the user must be shown to have: (1) had known about the risk before the incident, (2) voluntarily acted, and (3) unreasonably acted.

It should always be borne in mind that tampering or sabotage could have occurred to cause an accident. Tampering is defined as meddling for the purpose of altering, damaging, misusing, etc. Sabotage is malicious injury to work, tools, machinery, etc.

NEGLIGENCE

Negligence is the failure to conform one's conduct to that of a reasonable and prudent person. If such conduct results in harm to a person (or property) a lawsuit can be filed. The purpose of negligence law is protection from unreasonable risks or harm, which are foreseeable and therefore preventable. To prevail in a negligence lawsuit, four elements must be proven: (1) the existence of a duty of care, (2) breach of that duty, (3) proximate cause, and (4) damages establishment. The duty of care refers to behavior as a reasonable and prudent person; breach of that duty is obvious. Proximate cause refers to the value of personal injury, property damage, emotional stress, lost wages, etc. which resulted from the negligent behavior.

DESIGN DEFECT

A product does not have a design defect when it is safe for any reasonably foreseeable use. Such a safe product has also met all of the applicable functional specifications. Before a design defect can be alleged, it is necessary to establish that the product has met all applicable manufacturing, industrial, and governmental requirements, and despite meeting these requirements, the harmful incident occurred.

To establish that a design defect exists involves the following elements: (1) identification of the design defect, (2) establishing a link between the design defect and the harm done, (3) identification of alternate designs that would have prevented the harmful incident, and (4) comparing the product performance with like products offered by other manufacturers.

Perhaps a good example of a design defect is a product that functions normally under restricted circumstances. For example, if an apnea monitor operated properly in one environment, but failed to alarm cessation of breathing in another environment, the issue of design defect is raised. If the reason for failure were electromagnetic interference (EMI), it would be fruitful to inquire if similar apnea monitors provided by competitors also failed in the same environment or an equivalent environment. If they did not, it shows that there is technology available to eliminate this hazard. If the manufacturer of the monitor that failed was unaware, or chose to ignore the available technology, a case can be offered for design defect.

A disastrous case, which on first examination would appear like the failure of a life-support device, was described in the *South African Cape Times* (1996) which reported:

> For several months, our nurses have been baffled to find a dead patient in the same bed every Friday morning" a spokeswoman for the Pelonomi Hospital (Free State, South Africa) told reporters. "There was no apparent cause for any of the deaths, and extensive checks on the air conditioning system, and a search for possible bacterial infection, failed to reveal any clues.

Although device failure could cause such deaths, why they occurred on Fridays is difficult to understand. The hospital investigated further and the *Cape Times* reported:

> It seems that every Friday morning a cleaner would enter the ward, remove the plug that powered the patient's life support system, plug her floor polisher into the vacant socket, then go about her business. When she had finished her chores, she would plug the life support machine back in and leave, unaware that the patient was now dead. She could not, after all, hear the screams and eventual death rattle over the shirring of her polisher.
>
> We are sorry, and have sent a strong letter to the cleaner in question. Further, the Free State Health and Welfare Department is arranging for an electrician to fit an extra socket, so there should be no repetition of this incident. The inquiry is now closed.

The foregoing incidents raise many questions, such as "Shouldn't all life-support devices have loud alarms? Shouldn't all life-support devices have a backup battery supply? Why was there not a central monitoring station that exercised surveillance over all such patients?"

The issue of product design defect could well be raised because technology exists to prevent such deaths, either by alarming or provision of a built-in backup power supply. Any attorney involved in such a case would raise the issue of foreseeability, and would be correct in doing so. Finally, it may be appropriate to raise the issue of what minimal training should all have who are in an area where patients are on life-support equipment. Even a nonmedical person could sound an alarm or seek emergency assistance.

MEDICAL DEVICE REPORTS

In 1990, the U.S. Congress passed the Safe Medical Devices Act (SMDA), which went into effect on May 28, 1992 and was amended in 1995. This act and the amendments mandated the reporting of incidents associated with medical devices; such incidents must be reported to the FDA in the form of a Medical Device Report (MDR). Such MDRs are available from the FDA and can be useful in establishing facts in a lawsuit.

The most recent FDA regulation was published in the *Federal Register* of December 11, 1995 (21 CFR 803 and 807). This document clarifies and expands existing requirements for medical device manufacturers and health-care facilities. Failure to comply with this rule can result in increased risk of liability and civil penalty.

In February 1996, the Emergency Care Research Institute (ECRI) summarized the reporting requirements mandated by the Safe Medical Devices Act. The highlights of the reporting requirements are:

> Healthcare facilities must submit a report whenever they receive or otherwise become aware of information, from any source, that reasonably suggests that a device has or may have caused or contributed to a death or serious injury.
>
> The term "serious injury" is defined as an injury or illness that:
>
> 1. Is life threatening
> 2. Results in permanent impairment of a body function or permanent damage to a body structure or
> 3. Necessitates medical or surgical intervention to preclude permanent impairment of a body function or permanent damage to a body structure

Required to report are the following:

1. Hospitals, ambulatory surgical facilities, nursing homes, home-health agencies, ambulance providers, rescue groups, skilled nursing facilities, rehabilitation facilities, hospices, psychiatric facilities, and all other outpatient treatment and diagnostic facilities that are not a physician's office.
2. Manufacturers of medical devices
3. Distributors of medical devices (at present, covered by a different regulation)

Special forms are used to report device-related incidents. The report must be made within 10 working days of knowledge of the incident. MDRs are available from the FDA.

CHEMICAL HAZARDS

Sometimes an accident is associated with the use of a chemical compound or a substance classified as a drug. In such cases, valuable information can be found in the Materials Safety Data Sheet (MSDS), the Drug Insert (DI), and the Physician's Desk Reference (PDR); the address for the latter is P.O. Box 10689, Des Moines, IA, 50336-0689. The MSDS can be obtained directly from the manufacturer or the following:

Canadian Center for Occupation Health and Safety
CCOHS
250 Main Street, E.
Hamilton, Ontario, Canada L8N 1H6
1-800-668-4284

Genium Publishing Corp.
145 Catalyn Street
Schenectady, NY 12303
1-518-377-8854

The MSDS provides the correct name of the chemical substance, along with any synonym and brand name, the chemical composition, and physical and chemical properties. Fire, explosion, and health hazards are given, along with first-aid information. Reactivity and environmental factors, along with disposal techniques, are described. The sheet concludes with special precautions regarding use, storage, and handling procedures.

The Drug Insert is the data sheet that comes in the drug package; it lists indications, contraindications, side effects, toxicity, and antidotes. The PDR contains similar indicators and is indexed alphabetically by product name, product category, generic name, and chemical name. The PDR also provides an alphabetical listing of drug manufacturers.

The information provided by the sources identified may allow consideration of the foreseeability of the accident, the possibility of misuse, or uninformed use of a chemical substance.

THE INCIDENT REPORT

An incident report is a document that describes an event or events that caused harm, injury, or death to a patient. Such a report is composed at the time of or just after the incident by those present. The incident report does not assign culpability to anyone. On the contrary, it describes the incident in unambiguous language and often includes sketches showing the location of equipment and personnel. Healthcare facilities routinely complete and file incident reports, which are used by the institution to investigate the incident and promulgate rules or procedures to avoid such incidents. Because this document is composed by personnel on the scene at the time of the incident, it is very useful in contributing to an understanding of how the incident occurred. Incident reports are generally available to attorneys in a lawsuit. Over a 15-year period, I have been denied an incident report only once.

PRODUCT LIABILITY FUTURE

In the ideal world, the manufacturer provides a product that meets all applicable standards and is safe to use. It has been designed to avoid all foreseeable hazards in use and the instruction manual describes the intended purpose and use. The manual also contains a warranty, appropriate cautions, and warnings, along with information on service. There is no misrepresentation in the advertising. The vendor receives the product and conveys it to the customer in the same condition that it left the manufacturer's supervision. The manufacturer exercises a duty of due care to the customer.

The customer, who is a prudent and reasonable person, reads the instruction manual, then becomes a user of the product with safety and satisfaction. However, we live in a real world of rapidly expanding technology and a breakdown of one or more of the foregoing steps originates litigation.

It is likely that product development rate will exceed the recognition of foreseeable hazard, despite the regulatory requirements for inspection and testing. It often takes a long time for a defect to be revealed; it takes even longer to promulgate regulations that will eliminate the defect.

REFERENCES

AAMI (Association for the Advancement of Medical Instrumentation). 3330 Washington Blvd., Arlington, VA 22201-4598.
Althaus, J. *A Treatise on Medical Electricity.* 1873. Presley Blakiston, Philadelphia.
American National Standards Institute. 11 W. 42nd Street, New York 10036.
American Society for Quality Control. 161 West Wisconsin Avenue, Milwaukee, WI 53203.
Beard, G. M. and Rockwell, A.D. *On the Medical and Surgical Uses of Electricity.* 8th ed. 1891. W. Wood & Co., New York.
Canadian Standard Association. 235 Montreal Road, Ottawa 7, Ontario, Canada.
Capuano, M., Misole, P., and Davidson, D. Patient coupled device interaction produces arrhythmia-like artifact on electrocardiographs. *Biomed. Instr. Technol.* 1993, November–December: 475–483.
Department of Health and Human Services, FDA. Docket 91N-0295. *Federal Register* 1995, 60(237) December 11.
ECRI — Emergency Care Research Institute ECRI Advisory. February 1996. Safe Medical Devices Act. ECRI. 5200 Butler Pike Plymouth Meeting, PA 19462.
Enghagen, L.K. *Fundamentals of Product Liability Law for Engineers.* 1992, Industrial Press, Inc., New York.
Food and Drug Administration (FDA), Gaither Rd., MD 20850.

Geddes, L. A. A short history of electrical stimulation of excitable tissue including therapeutic applications. *Physiologist* (Suppl.) 1984, 22(1): S1–47.

International Electro Technical Commission (IEC). Centre du Service Clientele (CSC) Commission Electrotechnique Intenationale 3, rue do Varembe Case postale 131 CH1211, Geneve 20 (Geneva) Suisse (Switzerland).

National Electrical Code, National Fire Protection Association (NFPA). Battery Park, PO Box 9146, Quincy, MA 02269-9959.

Silberberg, J. What can/should we learn from reports of medical device electromagnetic interference?, at Electromagnetics, Health Care and Health, EMBS 95. September 19–20, 1995. Standards Promulgating Organizations, Montreal, Canada.

Underwriters' Laboratories, Inc. 207 East Ohio Street, Chicago, IL 60611.

U.S. Food and Drug Administration. Center for Devices and Radiological Health. 12720 Twinbrook Parkway, Rockville, MD 20857.

2 Electromagnetic Interference and Electrostatic Discharge

CONTENTS

INTRODUCTION

Electromagnetic interference (EMI) is the term used to describe malfunction of a device exposed to electromagnetic waves which have the property of propagating through space. That such high-frequency waves have this property was predicted by Maxwell in 1873. In 1888, Hertz demonstrated the accuracy of this prediction by generating them with a spark-gap transmitter. It was Marconi in 1903 who put this property to practical use to create wireless telegraphy, followed in 1906 by the first transmission of the human voice by Fessenden, both events giving rise to modern communications.

The frequency spectrum for electromagnetic waves ranges from the low-kilo-hertz range to thousands of gigahertz. The term hertz (Hz) replaced the old term "cycles/second". Table 1 identifies the terms used to designate the spectral bands. Various services are assigned to operate in these bands. In the U.S., the Federal Communications Commission issues the licenses to use the assigned frequencies. There are international treaties regarding the use of frequencies.

EMI is ubiquitous; the intensity is measured in volts/meter at a particular fre-quency. EMI is strongest in the urban areas where there is a plethora of communi-cations equipment. Bassen et al. (1992) stated:

TABLE 1
Frequency Allocations

Frequency Range	Designation
3–30 kHz	Very low frequency (VLF)
30–300 kHz	Low frequency (LF)
300–3000 kHz	Medium frequency (MF)
3–30 MHz	High frequency (HF)
30–300 MHz	Very high frequency (VHF)
300–3000 MHz	Ultrahigh frequency (UHF)
3–30 GHz	Super high frequency (SHF)
(1 GHz = 1000 MHz)	
30–300 GHz	Extremely high frequency (EHF)
300–3000 GHz	—

More than 1% of the U.S. population is exposed to ambient field strengths of more than 2 V/m by FM radio and VHF television broadcast transmitters operating in the 54 to 108 MHz frequency range. This information is especially significant in light of the existing requirements for RF susceptibility of medical devices. Present and proposed new EMC standards require immunity to field strengths of 1 to 3 V/m in this frequency range. Therefore, the effects of patient connection need to be accounted for in new medical device EMC standards. (EMC = electromagnetic compatibility.)

Medical devices can be influenced in many ways by electromagnetic radiation. Such devices can fail to operate or operate improperly, depending on the intensity, frequency, and type of modulation. EMI can be produced by communications equipment (radio, TV, cellular phones, pagers, etc.), arcing contacts, flashing lights, household appliances, video monitors, computers, electrosurgical and diathermy machines, etc. Those devices that produce intermittent bursts of EMI are the most troublesome; however, those that produce a constant level of EMI can also cause device malfunction by saturation.

It is not difficult to test a device for susceptibility to EMI. By such tests it can be determined to what frequency range it is sensitive and at what intensity (volts/meter). With this information, it is useful to determine if emitters producing this spectral range are in the environment, thereby making it possible to launch a fruitful investigation.

EMI can enter an electronic device by many different paths. For example, if the device is battery operated, EMI can gain easy access to electronic circuits if the cabinet housing it is unshielded. If a cable or a fluid-filled catheter connects the patient to the medical device, the patient and the connections can constitute an antenna. If the device is power-line operated, EMI can enter via the power line. If the device is battery operated and connected to a power-line-driven battery charger, EMI can enter via the power line.

TABLE 2
Broadcast Bands

Type	Frequency Range
Amplitude modulation (AM)	535–1605 kHz
Short wave (AM)	5.95–6.20 MHz
	9.50–9.775 MHz
	11.70–11.975 MHz
	15.10–15.45 MHz
	17.70–17.90 MHz
	21.45–21.75 MHz
	25.60–26.10 MHz
Frequency modulation (FM)	88–108 MHz
WWV standard time and frequency	5 MHz
	10 MHz
	15 MHz
	20 MHz
	25 MHz

SOURCES OF EMI

Any emitter of radiofrequency (electromagnetic) energy is a potential source of EMI. As stated previously, whether the source interferes or not depends on the frequency, type of modulation, intensity at the medical device, and its susceptibility. Various types of emitters are in the environment and the following identifies some of the more common types.

RADIO BROADCASTING

Although the first radio broadcasts used 50 and 100 kHz, the present amplitude modulation (AM) broadcast band extends from 535 to 1605 kHz. Below 535 kHz is reserved for navigational aids. There are numerous short-wave broadcast bands that employ AM; these are shown in Table 2. The frequency modulation (FM) broadcast band extends from 88 to 108 MHz; these data are summarized in Table 2 along with the frequencies used by WWV, which broadcasts standard time and frequency information day and night.

TELEVISION

The frequencies allocated for television broadcasting are shown in Table 3. The picture information is transmitted using amplitude modulation and the sound channels employ frequency modulation.

TABLE 3
Frequencies Assigned to the Television Channels

Channel No.	Band (MHz)	Channel No.	Band (MHz)	Channel No.	Band (MHz)
2	54–60	29	560–566	57	728–734
3	60–66	30	566–572	58	734–740
4	66–72	31	572–578	59	740–746
5	76–82	32	578–584	60	746–752
6	82–88	33	584–590	61	752–758
7	174–180	34	590–596	62	758–764
8	180–186	35	596–602	63	764–770
9	186–192	36	602–608	64	770–776
10	192–198	37	608–614	65	776–782
11	198–204	38	614–620	66	782–788
12	204–210	39	620–626	67	788–794
13	210–216	40	626–632	68	794–800
14	470–476	41	632–638	69	800–806
15	476–482	42	638–644	70	806–812
16	482–488	43	644–650	71	812–818
17	488–494	44	650–656	72	818–824
18	494–500	45	656–662	73	824–830
19	500–506	46	662–668	74	830–836
20	506–512	47	668–674	75	836–842
21	512–518	48	674–680	76	842–848
22	518–524	49	680–686	77	848–854
23	524–530	50	686–692	78	854–860
24	530–536	51	692–698	79	860–866
25	536–542	52	698–704	80	866–872
26	542–548	53	704–710	81	872–878
27	548–554	54	710–716	82	878–884
28	554–560	55	716–722	83	884–890
		56	722–728		

Data from International Telephone and Telegraph Corp. *Reference Data for Radio Engineers,* 5th ed., Howard W. Sams, Indianapolis, 1968.

PUBLIC SAFETY AND LAND TRANSPORTATION

The frequencies allocated to police, fire and emergency services, etc. are shown in Table 4. The frequency assigned to taxis, buses, trucks, railroads, etc. are shown in Table 5.

CELLULAR TELEPHONES AND PAGING SERVICES

Table 6 identifies the frequencies assigned to cellular telephones and Table 7 lists the frequencies assigned to wireless pagers.

TABLE 4
Public Safety (Police, Fire, Highway,
Forestry, and Emergency Services)

1605–1750	kHz
2107–2170	kHz
2194–2495	kHz
2505–2850	kHz
3.155–3.400	MHz
30.56–32.00	MHz
33.01–33.11	MHz
33.40–34.00	MHz
37.01–37.42	MHz
37.88–38.00	MHz
39.00–40.00	MHz
42.00–42.95	MHz
44.61–46.60	MHz
47.00–47.69	MHz
150.98–151.49	MHz
153.7325–154.46	MHz
154.6275–156.25	MHz
158.7–159.48	MHz
162.0–172.4	MHz
453.0–454.0	MHz
458.0–459.0	MHz

TABLE 5
Land Transportation
(Taxis, Trucks, Buses, Railroads)

MHz

30.56–32.00
33.00–33.01
43.68–44.61
150.8–150.98
152.24–152.48
157.45–157.74
159.48–161.575
452.0–453.0
457.0–458.0

AMATEUR RADIO AND CITIZENS BANDS

Table 8 identifies the frequencies assigned to amateur radio operators. Many different types of modulation are permitted in the amateur bands, providing the sidebands are limited to those specified by the FCC. Amateur radio operators require a license.

TABLE 6
Frequencies Assigned to Cellular Telephones

Cellular system A consists of 416 frequency pairs as follows:
    Mobile frequencies MHz
      824.040–834.990
      845.010–846.480
    Base frequencies MHz
      869.040–879.990
      890.010–891.480
Cellular system B consists of 416 frequency pairs as follows:
    Mobile frequencies MHz
      835.020–844.980
      846.510–848.970
    Base frequencies MHz
      880.020–889.980
      891.510–893.970
21 control-channel pairs are assigned to each cellular system: for system A, they are 834.390–834.990 and 879.390–879.990 MHz; for system B, they are 835.020–835.620 MHz.

Data from Bowker, J.D. *Electronic Communications Handbook,* Ingles, A.F., Ed., McGraw-Hill, New York, 1988.

TABLE 7
Wireless Paging Frequencies

Base Station Frequency, MHz	Paging Service
35.20–35.66	One way
43.20–43.66	One way
152.03–152.21	Two way for radio common carriers; mobile channels are spaced 6.46 MHz higher
152.51–152.81	Two way for wireline common carriers; mobile channels are spaced 5.26 MHz higher
454.025–454.350	Two way for radio common carriers; mobile channels are spaced 5.0 MHz higher
454.375–454.650	Two way for wireline common carriers; mobile channels are spaced 5.0 MHz higher

Data from Bowker. J.D. *Electronic Communications Handbook,* Ingles, A.F., Ed., McGraw-Hill, New York, 1988.

The frequencies allocated to personal communications are shown in Table 9. No license is required to operate in these frequency ranges, but the permissible power is limited.

INDUSTRIAL, SCIENTIFIC, AND MEDICAL

Radiofrequency current is used for a variety of purposes in industry and medicine and specific frequencies have been allocated for these uses; Table 10 identifies these

TABLE 8
Amateur Radio Frequencies

1800–2000 kHz
3.500–4.000 MHz
7.000–7.300 MHz
14.00–14.35 MHz
21.00–21.45 MHz
28.00–29.70 MHz
50.00–54.00 MHz
144.0–148.0 MHz
220.0–225.0 MHz
420.0–450.0 MHz
1215–1300 MHz
2300–2450 MHz
3.300–3.350 GHz
5.650–5.925 GHz
10.00–10.50 GHz
21.00–22.00 GHz
40.00–88.00 GHz
Above 90.00

TABLE 9
Citizens Radio
(Personal Radio Services)

MHz

26.96–27.23
462.525–467.475

frequencies. The lower frequencies (13.56 and 27.12 MHz) are used for short-wave diathermy in which body segments are heated. In some countries, 915 MHz is used for diathermy. Microwave diathermy uses 2450 MHz; this frequency is also used for microwave ovens.

It should be noted that electrosurgical units emit frequencies ranging from 0.5 to 2 MHz. This frequency range covers the standard AM broadcast band and there is no assigned frequency for this intermittent medical use.

RADAR

Radar employs repetitive short bursts of high-frequency electromagnetic radiation to locate the distance of a target using the pulse-echo technique. The frequencies used range from 3 MHz to 110 GHz, depending on the type of information sought.

TABLE 10
Industrial, Scientific,
and Medical Equipment

MHz

13.56
27.12
40.68 (government)
915.0 (government)
2450

However, frequencies from 1 to 100 GHz are common. The pulse repetition rate that can be used depends on the target distance. Electromagnetic waves travel in space at the rate of 186,000 mi/sec, i.e., 982 ft/μsec. Therefore, a target at a 982-ft distance would return an echo in 2 μsec. In general, the pulse repetition rate in most cases is low.

FREQUENCY, WAVELENGTH, AND ANTENNA EFFECT

The foregoing discussed the frequencies assigned to various services. Associated with frequency is wavelength, which in meters equals 300/frequency in MHz. The significance of wavelength becomes important when the length of the conductor becomes a fraction of one wavelength or more. One meter is equal to 39.4 in.

SKIN DEPTH

In a uniform conductor, direct current is distributed evenly over the cross section of the conductor. When sinusoidal alternating current flows in a uniform conductor, the current distribution becomes nonuniform, and as the frequency is increased, the current density at the perimeter increases. The term "skin depth" is used to quantitate this phenomenon and skin depth is that distance from the perimeter where the current density has fallen to 1/e, i.e., 37% of that at the surface. Skin depth (S) is calculated as follows:

$$S = \frac{1}{2\pi}\sqrt{\frac{10^9 \rho}{\mu f}}$$

where ρ is the resistivity (ohm-cm), μ is the permeability (1.0), and f is the frequency (Hz). Rearranging this expression yields:

$$S = 5028 \sqrt{\rho/f}$$

Note that the skin depth depends on the resistivity of the conductor and inversely with frequency. It is of more than passing interest to calculate skin depth for a metal, such as copper, and for biological material. Copper has a resistivity of 1.6×10^{-6}

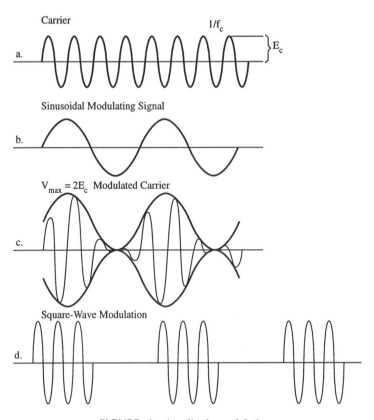

FIGURE 1 Amplitude modulation.

ohm-cm; therefore the skin depth in dentimeters is $6.36/\sqrt{f}$. Consequently, the skin depth is small in good conductors. In fact, high-frequency conductors are often made of tubing.

It is of interest to calculate the skin depth for tissue ($\rho = 500$ ohm-cm) exposed to a typical radar frequency (2.5×10^9 Hz). Entering these values into the skin-depth equation yields a skin depth of 2.25 cm.

MODULATION

Information is superimposed on a radiofrequency carrier and recovered at the receiving site. In general, there are two types of modulation: (1) amplitude and (2) frequency. Figure 1A illustrates an unmodulated carrier of frequency f_c and Figure 1B illustrates the signal that is to be applied to the carrier; Figure 1C illustrates the resulting 100% amplitude-modulated carrier. In this case, the peak amplitude of the modulated carrier is twice that of the unmodulated carrier. The modulation amplitude can range from 0 to 100%. At the receiving site, the modulation is stripped from the carrier.

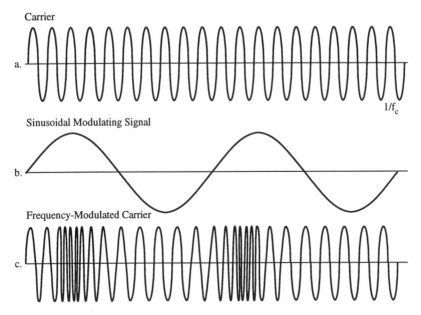

FIGURE 2   Frequency modulation.

Another type of amplitude modulation is shown in Figure 1D in which the carrier is turned on and off; this is the kind of signal used in wireless telegraphy and radar; Figure 1D represents the letter S in the Morse code (three dots). Of course the spacing and duration of the modulated carrier can be selected to conform to any desired coding scheme.

There is an inconsistency in modulation terms that arose with the passage of time. Originally a carrier that was modulated by the voice was designated wireless telephony. A carrier that was keyed on and off (Figure 1D) was called continuous wave (CW) by the radio amateurs and others. Nowadays continuous wave is used for an unmodulated carrier (Figure 1A).

Figure 2 illustrates frequency modulation of a carrier (A) by a sinusoidal modulating signal (B), resulting in the frequency-modulated carrier (C). In this case the frequency of the carrier is linearly related to the amplitude of the modulating signal, increasing and decreasing as the modulating signal goes positive, then negative. It should be obvious that if the modulating signal is a rectangular pulse, the carrier frequency will suddenly increase, then decrease. In all cases, the amplitude of the carrier is constant.

EXAMPLES OF DEVICE MALFUNCTION DUE TO EMI

The type of EMI produced by the various emitters of radiofrequency energy varies widely; those that are turned on and off are the most troublesome. For example, cellular and mobile telephones, paging systems, emergency services (ambulance, fire, and police), amateur radio, taxi radio, walkie-talkies, and several other types of communications are characterized by frequent, short periods of communication. Diathermy is turned on for about 20 to 30 min, whereas electrosurgical units are activated for only a few seconds each time cutting and/or coagulation are desired. Navigational devices vary widely in the type of radiofrequency signal that they emit; some operate at relatively low pulse frequencies, while others use high-frequency bursts of carrier. Those devices that emit bursts of radiofrequency energy can simulate heartbeats, respiration, brain-wave signals, or can even reprogram devices such as pacemakers, drug-delivery devices, ventilators, etc.

PATIENT SIMULATOR

EMI can be detected and interfere with devices connected to electrodes on a patient; examples of such are the EEG, EMG, ECG, impedance-based apnea monitors, etc. To investigate the susceptibility of such devices to EMI where they are used, it is practical to connect a patient simulator to the device. A simulator could be as simple as a resistor, or a calibrator that produces a known voltage or resistance change. The simulator should be capable of producing no signal as well as the signal appropriate for the device being tested. When the simulator is connected and no simulator signal is applied, the device should register no output; if it does, EMI is suspected. In the absence of a patient simulator, it is practical to use an easily created circuit, which, of course, produces no output, and when connected to the device, no signal will be registered in the absence of EMI.

ELECTRICAL EQUIVALENT FOR A SUBJECT

For a variety of reasons it is useful to have an electrical analog for the circuit formed when electrodes are placed on a subject. Such an analog (Z) evolved from 60-Hz leakage testing and it is sometimes called a patient dummy load or a patient simulator. The simplest equivalent for Z (Figure 3A) is a 500- or 1000-ohm resistor. The 500-ohm value was derived from the 60-Hz impedance of the body in good contact with ground. The 1000-ohm value was recommended by the National Fire Protection Association (NFPA, 76BM-3042).

The Association for the Advancement of Medical Instrumentation (AAMI) developed a standard circuit (Figure 3B), which exhibits a decreasing impedance with increasing frequency, as shown in Figure 4. At DC, the impedance is 1000 ohms; the impedance is very slightly less than 10 ohms at infinite frequency. The impedance at 60 Hz is a fraction of a percent below 1000 ohms.

Figure 3C illustrates the circuit recommended by the Canadian Standards Association (C 22.2, 1979). The impedance-frequency characteristic of this circuit is illustrated in Figure 4. The impedance decreases only slightly with frequency, starting out at 1000 ohms at 0 Hz and decreasing to 993 ohms at infinite frequency.

Not only are the circuits shown in Figure 3 useful for leakage-current testing, they are of value as a patient dummy connected to an ECG or impedance-respiration monitor. Because these three circuits are entirely passive — no output, i.e., a flat line will appear when connected to patient monitors. These equivalents do not apply when high current is applied to electrodes such as in defibrillation.

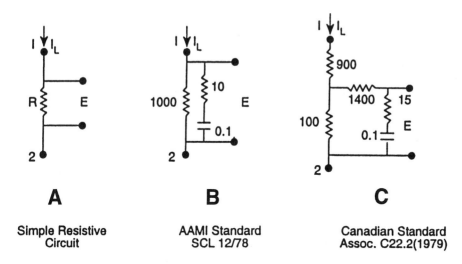

A

**Simple Resistive
Circuit**

B

**AAMI Standard
SCL 12/78**

C

**Canadian Standard
Assoc. C22.2(1979)**

FIGURE 3 Equivalent circuits for a pair of electrodes on a subject.

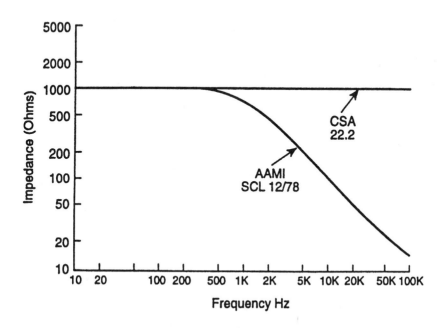

FIGURE 4 Impedance-frequency characteristics of the AAMI SCL 1278 and the CSA 22.2 equivalent circuits.

A saline filled, full-sized, plastic torso model of the body was described by Bassen et al. (1992). The model consisted of a plastic rectangular box (80 × 40 × 22 cm) with two cylindrical legs. Each leg had a diameter of 13 cm and a length of 86 cm. These legs were parallel to each other and attached to one end of the box in which 13-cm-diameter holes were cut. The model was originally developed for testing the susceptibility of pacemakers to electromagnetic pulses. Bassen et al. (1992) used the model to test the susceptibility of apnea monitors to EMI.

ELECTROENCEPHALOGRAPHIC   INTERFERENCE

Silbert et al. (1994) reported the first instance of EMI interference while recording the EEG. They stated:

> A four-year-old boy was referred to the Mayo Clinic EEG laboratory for evaluation of generalized tonic-colic seizures. The recording was performed on a 16-channel Grass electroencephalograph, using collodion application of electrodes, a high frequency filter of 70 Hz, a low frequency filter of 1 Hz, and a paper speed of 30 mm/sec. During the procedure both parents were present in the same recording room as the patient and the technologist. After approximately three minutes of recording, an unusual artifact appeared, which then recurred approximately every 40–120 seconds. The technologist was suspicious of an extrinsic electrical artifact, although no obvious source in the vicinity was apparent. She then asked the parents if they were carrying anything unusual. In fact, both had cellular telephones which were turned on, but had not rung or otherwise been used. Upon removal of the cellular telephones from the recording room to approximately 20 feet away, no further artifacts occurred. The recording, which demonstrated generalized epileptiform activity, was completed without further incident.

Silbert et al. carried out additional studies with different types of EEG machines using a Motorola DPC 550 cellular telephone. They stated that similar EEG artifacts were observed with other cellular telephones. They reported as follows:

> When the telephone was turned off, no artifact could be identified. When the telephone was turned on, but not otherwise being used, an "autonomous registration artifact" was seen recurring up to every 40 seconds. The artifact was present in several widely separated derivations (leads), varied in duration from 0.5–1.5 seconds, and was characterized by a series of spikes of 50 msec duration separated by 70–100 msec.

The foregoing demonstrates that when a cellular telephone is on and awaiting a call, it emits EMI (autonomous) pulses. In addition, pulses are emitted when the telephone is turned on and off. Also, as shown by Silbert et al., such spikes occurring in an EEG record could lead to misdiagnosis.

Additional information on the effects of EMI on medical devices due to cellular telephones will be presented elsewhere in this chapter.

ELECTROCARDIOGRAPHIC INTERFERENCE

ECG recordings are susceptible to EMI from a variety of sources, and the type of malfunction ranges from artifacts that resemble cardiac excitations to complete inhibition of the recording. The reporting sources range from investigative journalism to clinical engineering and medical records.

Writing in the *Wall Street Journal* on ECG malfunction, Knutson and Bulkeley (1994) reported:

> Michael Willingham, director of regulatory affairs for Physio-Control, says the radio waves were the source of the problem. He says company engineers discovered that the ambulance maker had replaced the metal roof of the vehicle with a fiberglass dome that didn't block radio waves well — then placed a powerful, long-range radio-transmission antenna atop it. Mr. Willingham says this is the only incident of its type involving LifePak (a defibrillator that contains an ECG).
>
> In 1992, a doctor installed an apparently unnecessary pacemaker in a patient's chest after an electrocardiogram telemetry system made by SpaceLabs Inc., also of Redmond, displayed "long periods of flat line." That evening, the same phenomenon recurred. Nurses discovered that the patient was next to a TV set when the flat line occurred. "Current labeling has warning about TV interference with telemetry signals," SpaceLabs reported to the FDA.
>
> "We've had only two or three instances of problems with EMI," says John Hall, vice president of quality assurance at SpaceLabs. "Another kind of diagnostic would normally be done" before implanting a pacemaker, he adds, but the company "can't tell people how to practice medicine."
>
> Physio-Control Corp., then an Eli Lilly Corp., Redmond, WA reported medical technicians taking a 93-year-old heart-attack victim to a hospital in 1991, attached her to one of the company's LifePak monitor/defibrillators to track and try to revive her failing heart. But they said the heart machine shut down every time the technicians turned on their radio transmitter. The woman died.

IMPEDANCE -BASED APNEA MONITOR MISHAPS

Many patient monitors use the small inspiratory-induced increase and decrease in transthoracic impedance to monitor respiratory rate. This technique was originally developed to monitor astronauts during spaceflight (Geddes et al., 1962). Typically, a low-intensity (e.g., 50 μA), high-frequency (10 to 100 kHz) current is applied to transchest electrodes, as shown in Figure 5. Because these electrodes are in an excellent location to detect the electrical activity of the heart, it is easy to obtain respiration and heart rate from the same pair of electrodes (Geddes et al., 1962). Figure 5 presents a record of these two events from the same pair of electrodes. Note the small rhythmic changes in heart rate with breathing. This normal event is called sinus arrhythmia. With slow breathing, heart rate increases slightly during inspiration and decreases slightly during expiration.

With apnea monitors, dry electrodes are usually employed and are located in a belt wrapped around the chest. The size of the impedance change depends on the

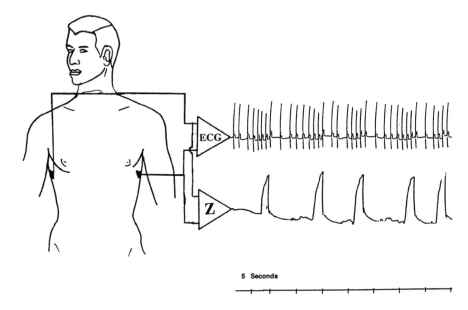

FIGURE 5 Method of obtaining the electrocardiogram (ECG) and impedance respiration (Z) from a pair of transchest electrodes.

size of the subject (Valentinuzzi et al., 1971). The maximum impedance change is obtained when the electrode pair is at about the level of the bottom of the sternum (xiphoid process). Dry electrodes, when first applied to the skin, exhibit a high impedance owing to the high skin resistance. This makes it difficult to obtain clean respiration and electrocardiac signals. Tap water or an electrode paste can be used to reduce the skin impedance. However, when a dry electrode is placed on the skin, perspiration can no longer evaporate from the site and with the passage of time, the skin becomes hydrated and the electrode impedance becomes less (Geddes and Valentinuzzi, 1973).

Impedance respiration and heart-rate monitors are appropriately band-pass filtered to accept these two signals. However, because the beating heart is between the transchest electrodes, there is a small pulsatile nonrespiratory (cardiac) signal in the respiration channel. Between breaths in Figure 5, these small cardiac impulses can be identified. To illustrate them better, Figure 6 is presented in which the recording sensitivity has been increased. In the center of the record, the subject stopped breathing and the cardiac impulses are clearly visible. Thus, with impedance respiration, cardiac impulses could be counted as breaths during apnea if the recording sensitivity is increased excessively. Such a condition could arise if the electrodes are not placed in the optimum location and the recording sensitivity is increased to detect breaths.

Monitor Alarms

All cardiorespiratory monitors are equipped with alarms that sound for a preset low and high heart rate and a preset low and high respiratory rate. Impedance and

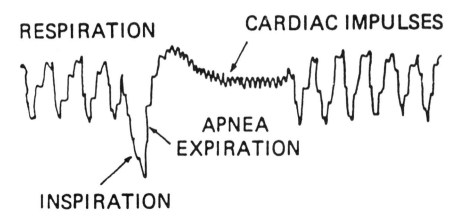

FIGURE 6 Impedance respiration during quiet breathing (left) and during apnea (center) showing cardiac impulses.

ECG-based monitors also have an electrodes-off (lead-off) alarm. These alarms are designed to alert the caregiver that the monitored patient needs prompt attention.

MECHANISM OF DEATH DUE TO APNEA

Respiration is neurogenic and the heartbeat is myogenic in origin. In other words, central nervous system integrity is needed for rhythmic breathing. No neurogenic activity is needed for the heartbeat because the heart's natural pacemaker (the S-A node) is in the heart — this is why transplanted hearts beat spontaneously.

A patient is usually placed on a cardiorespiratory monitor because there is a risk of respiratory arrest (apnea). If apnea occurs, the heart continues to beat and circulates blood with less and less oxygen. Very soon the oxygen delivery is inadequate and the heart rate gradually slows and ultimately stops beating.

If, in the scenario just described, the patient was connected to an impedance-based apnea monitor with the breathing sensitivity set high, the cardiac impulses could be counted as breaths and the breathing-rate alarm would fail to sound. The result would be increasing hypoxia (blueness) and likely brain damage and/or a failure to resuscitate when the low heart-rate alarm ultimately sounds.

To address the problem of counting a cardiac impedance impulse as a breath, Birnbaum and Stasz (1986) developed circuitry that sounds an alarm when the respiratory impedance-signal frequency was equal to the ECG heart-rate frequency. In the patent issued to them, it states:

> It is another object of the present invention to detect apparent heartbeat and respiration signals occurring at the same frequency and to generate an apnea alarm when such conditions exist.

SUSCEPTIBILITY TO EMI

Impedance-based apnea monitors, although designed to accept their own signals, are not immune from environmental EMI, the amount of which is increasing as new communications devices are introduced. Most existing apnea monitors were not designed to operate in areas where pulsating EMI signals are found. In fact, many ordinary devices emit EMI when turned on and off.

Ruggera and O'Bryan (1991) constructed a test chamber which provided controlled electromagnetic fields with frequencies ranging from 0.5 to 220 MHz. Into this chamber were placed several models of apnea monitors. The patient cable was connected to an ECG and breathing simulator, with the breathing signal inhibited. The field was 100% modulated at 0.5 Hz. Their study revealed that:

> EMI can cause disruption of apnea monitors at relatively low field strengths and at common communication frequencies. We also determined the field strength and frequency-dependent failure sensitivity of the monitors tested. The most sensitive model failed to alarm at a field strength below 0.1 V/m at a frequency in the FM broadcast band when 0.5 Hz 100% square-wave amplitude modulation was used.

Ruggera and O'Bryan carried out field-strength surveys in Washington, D.C., Omaha, NE, and Portland, OR, sites where apnea monitor failures had been reported. They stated:

> Some sites at which several of the monitors failed had high total field strengths, on the order of a few volts/meter. This supported laboratory findings that all monitors would fail when exposed to sufficient field strengths. A more typical situation at the survey sites was the existence of total RF field strengths of 0.4 to 1.0 V/m and "naturally occurring" modulation of the ambient fields. It was found that very low frequency amplitude modulation could be induced on RF fields at user sites by nearby moving objects such as people, pets, and cars. This produces time-varying multipath interference of the RF fields. Exposures to "moderate" strength RF fields that are intermittently amplitude modulated are potentially more of an EMI threat to apnea monitors than continual higher exposure since the former type of interference may be unsuspected.

It is important to note that the study by Ruggera and O'Bryan was published in 1991, when awareness to EMI was beginning to be recognized. However, apnea monitors made at that time are still in use and the need for EMI susceptibility testing is still present.

Ruggera et al. (1992) evaluated the susceptibility of nine impedance-based apnea monitors to EMI. They stated:

> Exposing the monitor to 100% square-wave modulated RF fields can cause the monitor to "think" it is sensing breath and/or ECG and not sound an alarm, even though no signals either from an infant or a patient simulator are being received.

Using a uniform radiofrequency field presented to the monitor, they stated:

> It was found that the fully extended (patient) leads became a much more effective receiver of RF interference over the frequency range of 10–53.5 MHz compared to earlier data taken in a TEM cell in the laboratory. Over this range the leads were approximately 0.1 to 0.5 wavelengths of the exposure frequency. An example of the

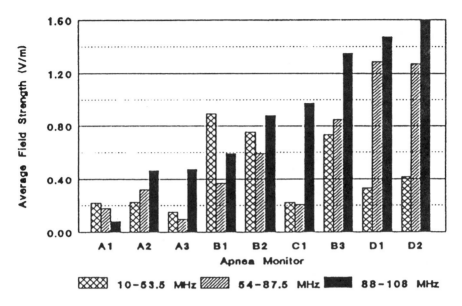

FIGURE 7 Field strengths for malfunction of nine apnea monitors. (Redrawn from Ruggera, P.S., O'Bryan, R., and Casamiento, J.P. Proc. IEEE EMBS Conf. 1992, 2839–2840.)

data obtained was presented as an EMI threshold field-strength vs. frequency plot from 1 to 220 MHz. Also, a field-strength average was calculated for three frequency bands in this range to summarize EMI threshold data for all nine of the apnea monitors tested. The high sensitivity of all monitors in a frequency band of 10 to 54 MHz used by CB radios, land-mobile communications, walkie-talkies, and amateur radio again emphasizes the need for the monitors to be hardened to withstand these common sources of ambient RF fields.

Figure 7 illustrates the EMI sensitivity of all nine monitors. Field strengths above the bars represent the values that will interfere with monitor operation.

Geddes (1995) investigated the susceptibility of three different impedance-respiration recorders, operating at 15, 35, and 45 kHz to EMI produced by arcing room thermostat contacts, a soldering gun, a hot-air gun, a fluorescent lamp, and electric hair clippers. Two types of tests were performed using (1) a loop antenna 2 ft in diameter with a 510-ohm resistor (dummy subject), shown in Figure 8A, and (2) a subject with transthoracic electrodes and a central ground (X), as shown in Figure 8B. The use of a ground (X) on the subject reduces the susceptibility to electrostatic discharge (ESD).

Figure 9A illustrates the output of an impedance recorder, operating at 33 kHz, connected to the loop antenna (Figure 8A) as the thermostat contact arced periodically. On the right is a 5-ohm calibration signal.

Figure 9B is a record of spontaneous respiration (left), breath holding (center), with transients from the thermostat during the 20-sec period of breath holding and the resumption of spontaneous breathing (right) in a subject monitored as in

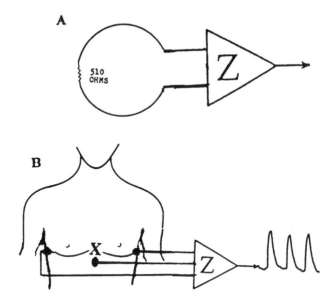

FIGURE 8 Impedance recording methods. A shows the impedance recorder (Z) connected to a 2-ft-diameter loop antenna with a 510-ohm resistor to simulate a subject. B shows the method used to record the respiratory-induced impedance change with transthoracic electrodes. The central electrode (X) serves to ground the subject to reduce susceptibility to electrostatic discharges.

Figure 8B at a distance of 2 ft from the thermostat. The small transient (T) during breath holding was produced by turning on the roof fluorescent lights.

Similar breath-size responses were obtained with the soldering gun, hot-air gun, fluorescent lights, and electric hair clipper.

Silberberg (1993), of the Center for Devices and Radiological Health (FDA), stated:

> Because there had been numerous reports of unexplained failure of apnea monitors to alarm upon death, the susceptibility of these monitors to radiated RF was evaluated by CDRH. After both laboratory and field testing, CDRH engineers determined that most commercial apnea monitors could erroneously detect respiration when exposed to relatively low field strengths, which could result in failure to alarm during apnea. Most monitors were found to be susceptible above 1 V/m when the field was pulsed or when an ambient FM field was incidentally amplitude modulated at a low rate of movement of objects and humans.
>
> One model was susceptible to pulsed fields above 0.05 V/m, and the manufacturer performed a recall to improve the immunity of its monitor, particularly in the FM broadcast band (88 to 108 MHz) … The same model was found to be unusually sensitive to quasi-static fields, detecting respiration when the monitor or cables were touched or when an electrostatically charged fabric was waved over the monitor.

Silberberg (1993) reported three other instances of mishaps with apnea monitors; he stated:

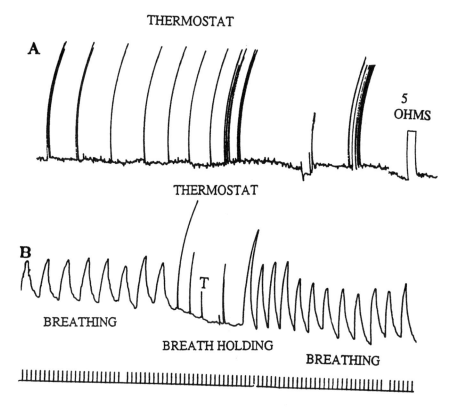

FIGURE 9   A shows the output of an impedance recorder operating at 33 kHz connected to the loop antenna (Figure 8A) placed 2 ft from arcing thermostat contacts. B shows spontaneous breathing (left) and breath holding (center), during which time the thermostat contacts were arcing. The transient T was produced when the room fluorescent lights were turned on. On the right, spontaneous breathing was resumed. (Time marks 1 sec.)

Neonatal monitors were interfered with when placed in close proximity to similar models of neonatal or adult monitors while operating in the shallow breathing mode at high gain.

Transmissions from an amateur radio station interfered with an infant monitor only when the remote alarm was attached.

A combination pulse oximeter and capnograph, which used a switching power supply with a frequency of 62.5 kHz, interfered with the impedance measurement circuit of respiration (apnea) monitors, resulting in false readings. The oximeter power supply frequency was close to the frequency used to measure transthoracic impedance in respiration monitors from three different manufacturers. The manufacturer of the pulse oximeter has issued a safety alert and will change the power supply frequency of the oximeters to prevent recurrence.

The foregoing indicates the need to test the susceptibility of apnea monitors for EMI at the site where used, by connecting a patient dummy load to the monitor which should show no breathing and sound the no-breathing alarm.

VENTILATOR MISHAPS

A ventilator is a device that inflates the lungs by providing intermittent air flow, usually delivered to an endotracheal tube; a tightly fitting face mask can also be used. The old name for a ventilator is a respirator. Because there is the need to control ventilation depth, rate, and the duration of inspiration, electronic controls are used, some of which can be quite sophisticated. Because such controllers are electronic, they are not immune from EMI.

Silberberg (1993) described a variety of ventilator mishaps due to EMI. He reported:

> A ventilator experienced keyboard lockup, due to interference from a guard's walkie-talkie.
>
> Two ventilators that were within 20 feet of each other alarmed simultaneously. That day the ventilators alarmed frequently; it was discovered that the power company was using walkie-talkies in the area. The hospital staff was able to duplicate the problem using walkie-talkies in the hospital.
>
> The operation of a particular model of ventilator was disrupted, resulting in cessation of ventilation, inoperative monitoring functions, display or error messages, or display of unintelligible messages. The disruptions were caused by "extreme events" of EMI or power-line disturbances, possibly resulting from the use of electrosurgical, laser, X-ray, or other equipment.
>
> A ventilator went into "safety valve open" and displayed an error code during a chest X-ray.
>
> A microprocessor-based intensive care ventilator ceased operating and alarmed, and microprocessor-based infusion pumps stopped working when a portable X-ray machine was turned off in the vicinity.
>
> The operation and readouts of ventilators were affected by keying of two-way hand-held FM radios, both in the same room and in the next room. The low minute volume alarm would sound, the analog display would indicate an exhaled minute volume of zero, and the digital display would indicate negative values of exhaled minute volume.
>
> Four-watt walkie-talkies used for communication within a hospital interfered with the operation of high-frequency ventilators up to a distance of 10 feet, causing the bar graph display of piston location and amplitude to be driven out of the display window, and the pressure readout to decrease enough to trip low pressure alarms, which caused the piston to stop. The manufacturer found that replacing the plastic cover of the electronic control assembly with a metal cover would result in only a 2-cm error in the displayed mean pressure and no error in the actual delivered mean pressure.
>
> RF transmission from a hospital source (hand-held two-way radio) or an outside source caused a ventilator to activate alarms. The hospital was able to duplicate the event.
>
> While in use during a flight, a portable ventilator operating on battery power stopped cycling and alarmed several times. Factory evaluation revealed that radio frequency interference caused false signals. The unit was updated and the cable was shielded.

DRUG-INFUSION PUMP MISHAPS

Drugs are often injected into the vascular system via a programmable infusion pump. Typically, a sterile syringe containing the drug is inserted into the pump and the delivery program is entered by a keyboard. Such devices are typically microprocessor controlled and can be susceptible to EMI.

Silberberg (1993) cited the following cases of infusion-pump malfunction; he reported:

> An infusion pump changed rate when a cellular phone was placed on the instrument stand.
> An infusion device on an isolated circuit (high source impedance) behaved erratically due to conducted EMI at 33 MHz.

POWERED-VEHICLE MISHAPS

Motor-driven wheelchairs and scooters used by patients contain electronic controls which have malfunctioned in the presence of electromagnetic radiation. Silberberg (1993) reported:

> A quality assurance manager who had previously worked for a large wheelchair manufacturer, in a letter dated June 26, 1992, inquired about the status of medical device EMC standards. As a side issue, he reported that in his previous position he had received reports of powered wheelchairs driving off curbs and piers unintentionally when a police or fire vehicle, harbor patrol boat, or CB or amateur radio was in the vicinity. The reporter had reproduced the phenomenon under controlled conditions and had observed powered wheelchairs "go by themselves" within 15 or 20 feet of a police or firetruck radio. (EMC = electromagnetic compatibility.)
>
> The CDRH databases were checked for reports of electromagnetic interference problems with powered wheelchairs. While several reports of unintended motion were found, several involving serious injury, none had been attributed to electromagnetic interference in the report.
>
> CDRH engineers investigated the EMI susceptibility of the motion controllers of several makes of powered wheelchairs and scooters. The powered wheelchairs tested were found to be susceptible to field strengths in the range of 5 to 15 V/m. At the lower end of the susceptibility range, the electric brakes would release, which could result in a hazard of rolling if the chair were stopped on an incline. As the field strength at a susceptible frequency was increased, the wheels would begin turning, with the speed of rotation a function of the field strength.
>
> CDRH engineers also measured the emissions from police and fire radios. A 100-watt state police radio transmitting at 39 MHz was found to have a field strength of 41 V/m at a distance of 0.9 m. CDRH also learned that a small number of manufacturers of wheelchair controllers supply much of the powered wheelchair and scooter industry.

Further studies on the effect of EMI on wheelchairs were reported by Witters (1995), who stated that the FDA became aware of this problem in 1992 and launched a susceptibility investigation over the frequency range from 50 to 90 MHz. He stated that the wheel speed was measured over a range of field strengths. For these tests, the wheelchair controller was turned on with the 'joystick' in the neutral position (wheelchair stationary). The wheel speed was monitored in revolutions per minute (rpm). If there were no EMI-induced movements, the wheels would have remained stationary at 0 rpm. In this case the wheels were induced to move at several different speeds, some quite fast.

He stated: "One of the main observations made was that the device would react differently for the different field strength levels of EM energy, creating windows of effects." He concluded:

> The CDRH laboratory results clearly indicated an EMI problem for these devices. Further testing revealed that the EMI seemed to affect the control system of the powered wheelchairs. In many cases, motorized scooters utilize the same type of control systems, thus there was concern for EMI with these devices. Testing indicated the scooter devices could exhibit EMI problems.

CELLULAR AND MOBILE TELEPHONE -GENERATED EMI

It is estimated that there are 16 million cellular telephones in use in the U.S. at present. Bren (1996) estimated that by the end of the 1990s, there will be over 60 million users nationally. With this tremendous expansion in service, the opportunity for interaction with medical devices will increase dramatically. At present there are two technologies employed: analog and digital. In the U.S., the NATEL-C system employs frequency modulation operating in the 824- to 849- and 869- to 894-MHz bands. It is important to note that even when the cellular telephone is not being used (but turned on), it emits signals that are identified by the base station. The method used in Europe is digital and is designated GSM (Global Standards for Mobile Communication), which emits 8/sec pulses in the 890- to 915-MHz band for signal transmission to the base station and in the 935- to 960-MHz band from the base station. Two types of digital phones are being introduced in the U.S., one is called Code Division Multiple Access (CDMA) and the other is designated Time Division Multiple Access (TDMA); this latter technology is similar to that used in the GSM. Therefore, when investigating the performance of medical devices exposed to electromagnetic radiation emitted by cellular telephones, it is essential to identify the type of technology used by the telephone.

Infant Radiant Warmer Mishaps

An AAMI (1996) committee is drafting a list of incidents in which EMI has caused dysfunction in medical devices. One entry in this preliminary report states:

> On December 1, 1994, the television program *Eye to Eye with Connie Chung* aired a story on the EMI effects of wireless transmitting devices on medical devices. In January 1995, at a hospital in the Southwest, testing was performed in an effort to duplicate the effects reported on the program. The testing involved a similar type of

infant radiant warmer and its response to an imposed electromagnetic field produced by (1) a hand-held transceiver and (2) a cellular telephone. It was found that the hand-held transceiver affected the infant warmer at distances up to 10 feet away, depending on the transceiver's battery charge. The cellular telephone affected the device only if it was located within 18 inches of the infant radiant warmer.

The report concludes by stating:

> As a result of these tests and others performed on infusion pumps, PCA pumps, infant ventilators, and certain monitors, the Safety Committee decided, upon recommendation by the Clinical Engineering Department, to restrict the use of hand-held transceivers and cellular telephones in the critical care, labor and delivery, nursery, respiratory care, EEG, EMG, and cardiology areas of the hospital. (Hand-held transceivers can be used to receive in those areas, but can be used to transmit only in unrestricted areas. Cellular telephones must be turned off.) Memos and letters were sent to physicians and to the directors of the affected departments to explain the need for the restrictions. Videos were presented to the Safety Committee to provide evidence of the interactions between hand-held transceivers, cellular telephones, and medical devices.

Clifford et al. (1994) investigated the effect of several mobile, hand-held telephones on nearby medical devices. The study was performed in Australia using two different types of telephones: (1) Advanced Mobile Phone System (AMPS) and (2) Global System Mobile (GSM). The AMPS is an analog FM communication system operating between 825 and 845 MHz with a power of 0.6 W. The GSM is a digital communication system that operates in the 890- to 915-MHz band with 0.6-msec pulses having a repetition rate of 217 Hz. The output power ranged from 0.8 to 2 W. Hand-held telephones of both types were brought close to the following medical devices: two patient monitors, six drug-infusion pumps, a defibrillator monitor, a cardiac monitor, a pulse oximeter, an oxygen monitor, a blood-pressure monitor, a fetal monitor with telemetry, and an ECG telemeter. They stated their results as follows:

> The AMPS phone operating at 0.6 W affected only three pieces of equipment: the ECG trace was distorted on one of the patient monitors and two of the pumps initiated false alarms, though one of these pumps gave false alarms only when the antenna of the phone was within 50 mm of its case. This result suggests that manufacturers have generally adhered to the FDA standard and hardened their equipment to withstand fields of 7 V/m or greater.
>
> When the same pieces of equipment were tested with the (digital) GSM phones seven of them operated normally. The other eight displayed the following symptoms: distortion or loss of ECG traces, false alarms and halting/change of speed of infusion pumps, and the introduction of severe distortion into the telemetry systems, including a 217 Hz audible interference tone on one unit. Increasing the power of the GSM phone did not change the symptoms, except in one case when the higher power phone triggered an alarm in addition to the other symptoms. Changing from the 2-W phone to the 8-W model doubled the distance within which interference effects were observed.

Three of the pumps were not affected at all, and at distances greater than 200 mm, the other three were free from interference even from the 8-W phone. Within the critical distances, the three pumps displayed various error messages; two of them then ceased to operate and one continued to operate but at two-thirds of its selected rate.

The ECG display in the defibrillator/monitor was free of interference, but the other three units with ECG monitors displayed a variety of symptoms including blanking of one CRT unit and/or horizontal lines, and high levels of noise on the ECG trace which initiated alarms in two of the units. In one of the units the distortion persisted at distances up to 2 m with the 8-W phone.

The pulse oximeter unit in one of the patient monitors showed a low signal at distances up to 2 m with the 8-W phone.

Both telemetry systems were affected by the GSM phones producing interference and large excursions of the trace. One unit had a 217-Hz interference which was audible. No interference was observed when the phones were more than 2 m from both the transmitters and the receivers.

Of considerable value in the Clifford paper is a tabulation of the peak field strength (volts/meter) at different distances from the 0.6- and 2-W hand-held telephones. These data are plotted in Figure 10. Although there is no universally accepted standard for the maximum permissible field strengths at different distances, Clifford et al. (1994) stated:

It is our concern that the existing 1979 FDA standard can be exceeded at distances of up to 2 m with an 8-watt transportable digital phone. The clear implication of this result is that digital phones will cause more EMI than the current analogue phones; this was confirmed in the interference tests with selected medical electrical equipment. It is also of concern that the IEC have set a less stringent standard, i.e., 3 V/m, than the FDA's 7 V/m.

Additional field-strength data for hand-held cellular phones (0.6 W) and transceivers (5 W) were reported by Foster (1994). Table 11 lists the range of distances from a series of these instruments for field strengths of 1 and 3 V/m.

Bostrom (1991) reviewed a series of European incidents involving mobile telephones and medical devices. He stated:

One of the first reports was from Denmark, where a single-patient haemodialysis monitor stopped working when a mobile telephone was used on the floor under the dialysis department. In another case a dialysis monitor malfunctioned in Sweden when a patient used his own mobile telephone during dialysis in a hospital. The patient noticed the alarm from the monitor and stopped using his telephone. The incidence of malfunction then ceased.

Several problems with different kinds of electromedical equipment in Norway have been reported in *Hyhetsrevy,* which is a Norwegian newsletter about accidents and incidents with medical devices published by the Norwegian Institute for Hospital Research in Trondheim. Incubators, syringe infusion pumps, infusion controllers, dialysis equipment, and defibrillators have been reported to malfunction due to interference from mobile telephones.

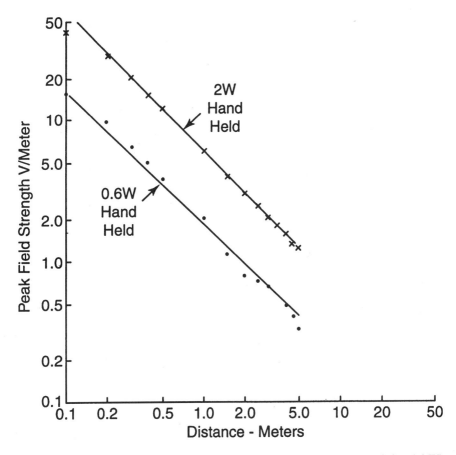

FIGURE 10 Field strength (V/m) vs. distance (m) for hand-held phones (0.6 and 2 W). (Data from Clifford, K.J., Joyner, K.H., Stroud, D.B., et al. *Austral. Phys. Eng. Sci. Med.* 1994, 17(1): 23–27.)

TABLE 11
Distance from Personal Communications
Devices for Field Strengths of 1 and 3 V/m

Instrument Type	Distance[a] 1 V/m	In Feet for 3 V/m
Cellular phone (0.6 Watts)	1–8	0.5–3
Transceiver	3–25	1–8

[a] Expected range for different units.

Data from Foster, K. *Sci. Eng. Biomed.* 1994, December.

So far only a few incidents have been documented, but some of them have been rather serious. In one case a home patient's lung ventilator changed its function in a serious way; in another case an infusion pump, used for administration of a potent drug, switched to the maximum infusion speed. I have been told that the death of a patient due to electromagnetic interference with an infusion pump has occurred in Japan. But since no report about this accident has been written in English it has not been possible for me to check the circumstances of that specific case.

Bostrom concluded by stating:

Many hospitals in the Scandinavian countries have now prohibited the use of mobile telephones (and radio transmitters) within the whole hospital area. Other hospitals have prohibited the use of such equipment only in certain zones with susceptible electromedical devices, e.g., intensive care units, operating theatres, and dialysis departments. Still other hospitals have only informed the medical staff and clinical engineers about the risks and warned about the use of mobile telephones within certain distances (e.g., 5 m) from electromedical devices. The nations' authorities for health and welfare in Sweden, Norway, and Finland have also sent out alerts with information about the safety risks with mobile telephones.

Health Effects

Because cellular phones are held close to the head, some concern has been raised about potential health effects. The research to date was summarized by Bren (1996), who stated:

Thus far, no supportable evidence has been brought forth to show that exposure to non-ionizing radiation from cellular telephones causes adverse health effects.

PAGING SYSTEM -GENERATED EMI

Paging systems vary in output power considerably and are capable of causing medical devices to malfunction. Silberberg (1993) reported the following incidents:

The reading of all invasive blood pressure monitors in an ICU/CCU jumped 3 to 10 mm Hg when a 150-W paging transmitter on the hospital roof was activated.
Displays of a telemetry patient monitor would "flat-line" when a paging company transmitted digital control information to its remote sites.

CARDIAC PACEMAKERS AND EMI

INTRODUCTION

There are three types of cardiac pacemakers: (1) external, (2) temporary, and (3) implanted. The external type delivers pulses (20 to 40 msec) to transchest electrodes. The temporary type delivers pulses (<1 msec) to a catheter electrode passed down a vein into the right ventricle. The implanted type is contained in a metal enclosure (can), usually implanted in the chest, and delivers its pulses to the heart via a catheter electrode.

CLOSED -CHEST CARDIAC PACEMAKERS

Cardiac pacing with chest-surface electrodes was introduced by Zoll (1952). Because transient cardiac arrest and/or atrioventricular block follows ventricular defibrillation, many of the early transchest defibrillators included a pacemaker. However, because the shocks used then were so unpleasant to the subject, these pacemakers were not included in later defibrillators. Zoll et al. (1981) found that by using a long-duration pacing pulse (20 to 40 msec), large-area electrodes, and a high-resistivity gel under the electrode, the skin sensation was markedly reduced. By mid-1982 closed-chest cardiac pacemakers became available commercially using self-adhering disposable electrodes (about 100 cm^2), long-duration pulses (20 to 40 msec), and a peak current of 60 to 100 mA. The high-resistivity gel reduces high-peak current density that is prominent under the perimeter of an electrode that uses a low-resistivity coupling agent. Typical pacing rates are 70/min and above.

To date the author has found no reports of malfunction of a closed-chest pacemaker due to EMI. However, there are reports of complications associated with long-term closed-chest pacing. For example, skin damage under the electrodes has been observed in human subjects when pacing has been applied for more than 8 h. For this reason some manufacturers place a pacing-time limit instruction on the electrodes.

A full-thickness skin injury due to prolonged closed-chest pacing (45 h) of a 7-week old child was reported by Pride and McKinley (1990). The pacing electrodes were designed for use on children less than 15 kg. In commenting on the electrodes, they stated: "Due to the child's very small chest there was little surface area available for the pacing pads."

After 45 h of pacing at 80 to 85 pulses per minute with a current of 40 to 60 mA, they reported: "When the pads were removed, a large bullous second-degree burn was noticed on the back. A 3-cm eschar covering a full-thickness burn penetrating to the pectoralis muscle was found anteriorly." Thus, injury occurred under both electrodes, but the degree of injury was slightly different.

It is of value to calculate the average current that flowed. Typically, the duration of a transchest pacing pulse is 25 msec. The total number of pulses delivered when pacing at 80 to 85/min for 45 h is 45×60 (80 to 85) = 216,000 to 229,500 pulses. Each pulse is typically 25 msec; therefore, the equivalent duration of current flow is 25×10^{-3} (216,000 to 229,500), which is equal to 5400 to 5737 sec.

The charge transferred describes the electrolytic process at the electrode interface and is equal to the product of current and time. In this case, the pacing current was 40 to 60 mA; therefore, the range of charge was 5400×40 = 216,000 to 5737 $\times$ 60 = 344,200 mA-sec or 216 to 344 C (amp-sec). Clearly, this amount of charge produced skin lesions.

A high electrode current density, persisting for a long time, can cause tissue injury. In this case, it is not possible to calculate the current density accurately; but if the 3-cm lesion is taken as the effective electrode diameter, the current density is the current divided by the electrode area. In this case, the estimated current density is 40 to 60 mA divided by $0.785 \times 3 \times 3$ cm^2, or a current density range of 5.67 to 8.50 mA/cm^2. It is clear that this current density, when applied for 45 h at a pacing rate of 80 to 85/min, produced skin lesions.

Pride and McKinley (1990) pointed out that "In contrast to adult skin, neonatal skin is thinner, has less hair, weaker intracellular attachments, fewer eccrine and sebaceous gland secretions and an increased susceptibility to external irritants." These factors may have contributed to the severity of the lesions.

In the introduction to their paper, Price and McKinley (1990) stated that "after having received reports of burns during prolonged pacer use in neonates, the ZMI Corporation has issued a warning that pacing for 1 to 2 h may cause thermal injury and that skin should be inspected every 30 min (unpublished FDA report distributed by Zoll, February 1988)."

The nature of the skin lesions described by Pride and McKinley (1990) merits speculation regarding their possible cause. Note that the injury under the two electrodes was different, despite the fact that they both carried the same pacing current. If one electrode skin-contact area were smaller than the other, the current densities would be different and therefore the severity of the lesions would be different. The lesion on the back was decribed as "a large bullous second-degree burn;" a bullous is a blister filled with serous fluid. The lesion on the chest was "a 3-cm eschar covering a full-thickness burn penetrating to the pectoralis muscle;" an eschar is dead tissue cast off living tissue produced by burning or the application of a corrosive substance. Thus, the severity of the chest lesion was greater than that on the back despite the same total current flow at each site. However, we do not know the contact areas at both sites.

It was not proven that the "burn" was thermal in origin. The term "burn" is also used for chemical injury and it is logical to speculate on this point. When unidirectional (pulses or continuous) current flows through an electrode coupled to the skin via an electrolyte, local chemical injury can result from electrolysis of the electrolytic coupling agent, which is predominantly an aqueous solution of sodium chloride that provides Na^+, Cl^-, H^+, and OH^- ions. With a unidirectional current pulse, one electrode becomes positive and the other negative. Negatively charged ions (Cl^- and OH^-) are attracted to the positive electrode and positively charged ions (Na^+ and H^+) are attracted to the negative electrode and a variety of chemical reactions can occur. For example, gaseous oxygen, hydrogen, and chlorine can be liberated. Gaseous chlorine is soluble and is a strong bleaching agent. Sodium is a corrosive element which can combine with hydroxyl ions to form sodium hydroxide, which is corrosive to all tissues. The hydrogen ions can combine with the chloride ions to form hydrochloric acid, a corrosive agent. In general, the environment of the negative electrode is acidic and that of the positive electrode is basic. This fact is easily proven by applying litmus paper at each site and noting the nature of the color change. Beyond these chemical compounds are those that may be formed by the material of the electrodes. Because one electrode is positive and one is negative, the chemical products at each are expected to be different and therefore the lesions are expected to be different. As yet, there has been no study that has quantitated the type of skin damage under the positive and negative electrodes having the same area carrying the same current.

Iontophoresis is another mechanism which could participate in skin damage when unidirectional current is passed through an electrode–skin interface. Iontophoresis is the process by which direct current is used to drive a charged substance into the skin. Typically, the material to be transported is enclosed in a cup-shaped electrode applied to the skin. A large area, distant indifferent electrode completes the circuit. If the substance to be driven through the skin has a positive charge, the electrode in the cup is made positive. The opposite applies for negatively charged substances. Typically, a current density of less than 2 mA/cm^2 is used. By identifying the charge on the substances in the electrolyte used with an electrode, and knowing the electrode polarity, it is possible to predict which substances will be driven through the skin. More details on iontophoresis appear in the chapter on direct-current injury.

Implanted Pacemakers

There are many reports of implanted pacemaker malfunction due to EMI and the following paragraphs will provide illustrative examples. It should be noted that several different types of malfunction can occur. For example, a pacemaker exposed to EMI may be inhibited and fail to deliver cardiac-pacing stimuli. It may revert to the fixed (constant)-rate pacing mode; it may be triggered to produce rapid pacing or even cause ventricular fibrillation. The internal program may be reset to an inappropriate pacing mode. Finally, a pacemaker may be destroyed and cease to produce pacing stimuli.

Pacemaker manufacturers issue warnings against the use of pacemakers in the vicinity of radiofrequency generators. Before describing pacemaker malfunctions it is useful to discuss the normal function of the heart.

The Cardiac Cycle

The origin of the heartbeat in a normal subject is in the sinoatrial (S-A) node, located in the upper right atrium (Figure 11). This region of modified cardiac muscle is really a chemical oscillator that has the interesting property of developing rhythmic electrical activity which is propagated to the atria, causing them to contract and pump blood into the ventricles. The wave of propagated excitation, represented by the P wave of the ECG, travels over the atria and reaches the atrioventricular (A-V) node in the base of the right ventricle. The propagation velocity of excitation through the A-V node is slow; therefore, there is a delay in propagating excitation to the ventricles, thereby allowing them to fill. Excitation leaving the A-V node is propagated along the bundle of His and Purkinje fibers, ultimately arriving at the ventricular muscle, giving rise to the QRS wave, after which the ventricles contract. This arborizing network of fibers is called the conduction system, which serves to coordinate the spread of excitation so that a forceful ventricular beat ensues, thereby pumping blood from the ventricles. Relaxation of the ventricles is preceded by the T wave of the ECG; Figure 11 shows a complete electrical cycle of the heart (P, QRS, and T).

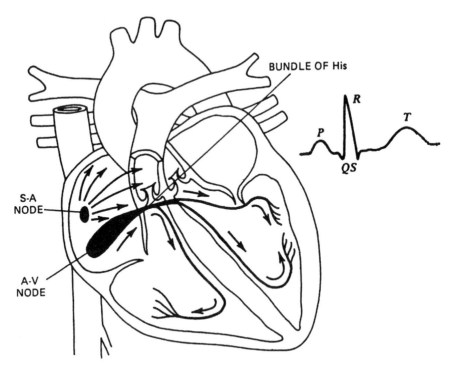

FIGURE 11 The pathways traversed by excitation that gives rise to atrial contraction and then ventricular contraction. In the normal heart, the sinoatrial (S-A) node is the pacemaker; the atrioventricular (A-V) node propagates excitation via the bundle of His and Purkinje fibers to the ventricular muscle.

Normally the rate of the heart is determined by the rhythmicity of the S-A node. It is important to emphasize that the S-A node is spontaneously rhythmic. An excised heart will continue to beat for some time. The rhythmicity of the S-A node is influenced by temperature, nervous, and chemical (humoral) activity. Increasing temperature and an increase activity of the sympathetic nervous system increase the heart rate and force of ventricular contraction, thereby increasing blood pressure and cardiac output. Increase activity of the parasympathetic nervous system decreases the heart rate, thereby decreasing blood pressure and cardiac output. These two branches of the autonomic nervous system are controlled by centers in the medulla and hypothalamus.

While it is true that under normal circumstances the heart rate is dependent on the activity of the S-A node, other areas in the heart can become pacemakers and originate a heartbeat. Atrial muscle fibers, the A-V node, the ventricular conducting system, and ventricular muscle fibers all have the capability of becoming rhythmic and acting as pacemakers. For this reason, it is possible that the heartbeat may not always consist of an orderly sequence of atrial contraction followed by ventricular contraction. In A-V block, the ventricles can become spontaneously active and beat rhythmically with no relation to atrial contractions. However, when this situation

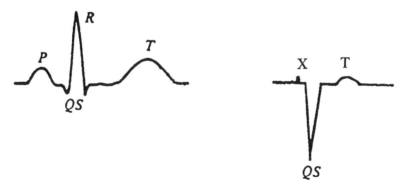

FIGURE 12   Normal ECG (A) and (B) the ECG in response to a pacing stimulus X.

arises, the ventricular rate is usually so slow that an inadequate cardiac output results and a pacemaker is needed.

Advancing age and disease can disrupt the organization of the heartbeat. One of the most important cardiac impairments is atrioventricular (A-V) block. In this situation, the rhythmic excitations of the atria are not propagated through the A-V node. Sometimes two, three, or more atrial excitations occur before one ventricular beat occurs; this situation is called partial or second-degree A-V block. In many circumstances, none of the atrial excitations pass beyond the A-V node and the ventricles are thereby deprived of their normal pacemaker drive. In this situation, which is called total or third-degree A-V block, the most rhythmic region in the ventricles will start pacemaking and develop propagated excitation that will travel throughout both ventricles. However, in such a case the ventricular rate is often too slow to provide adequate cardiac output for consciousness or normal activity. Rhythmic stimulation of the ventricles by a cardiac pacemaker can provide adequate cardiac output.

From the foregoing it can be seen that although the atria and ventricles may lose their pacemaking drive, they can be made to contract by an electrical stimulus provided by a cardiac pacemaker. Thus, atrial or ventricular, or atrial and ventricular stimulation can be applied to restore cardiac output to a level compatible with the maintenance of a reasonable quality of life.

When an electronic pacemaker is used to evoke cardiac contractions, the ECG is different from that in a normal subject. For example, the pacemaker stimulus can be identified in the ECG as a spike followed by the wave of excitation that it produces. For example, Figure 12A shows a normal ECG, consisting of the P, QRS, and T waves. Figure 12B shows ventricular pacing; X identifies the pacing stimulus, followed by the ventricular QS-T complex.

THREE -LETTER CODE

A three-letter code has been adopted to designate the type of pacemaker. The first letter identifies the chamber that is paced, that is, atrium (A) or ventricle (V) or doubly (D). The second letter identifies the chamber sensed (A,V, D), and the third letter specifies the mode of operation, I being used to identify inhibited and T designating triggered. The letter O is used to identify that a particular descriptor is inapplicable. For example, the original (asynchronous), fixed-rate ventricular pacemaker would be designated VOO. The popular ventricular-demand pacemaker is identified by the letters VVI to specify that the pacemaker is inhibited by activity. A fourth letter R is used to identify rate sensitivity, i.e., the pacing rate increases in response to activity.

COMMUNICATION WITH AN IMPLANTED PACEMAKER

Two-way telemetry is possible between an implanted pacemaker and the programmer that is placed on the skin above the implant. The programmer can interrogate the pacing parameters, pulse current, duration, rate, battery voltage, electrode impedance, etc. The programmer can also set the mode of operation of the pacer. In addition, a magnet placed on the skin above the pacer can revert the pacer to another mode. This technique is used to identify the pacing rate which is indicative of battery voltage and thereby identify when pacemaker replacement is needed.

EFFECT OF EMI ON PACEMAKER FUNCTION

In reviewing the literature on the effect of EMI on cardiac pacemakers, it is important to recognize that the early units were not designed to reject EMI. Serious attention to the effects of EMI on pacemakers was slow to evolve and it is difficult to specify a date when improvements were made to attenuate this problem. However, an editorial by Furman (1982) provides insight; he wrote:

> It has been recognized for at least two decades that electromagnetic signals exist which can interfere with pacemaker function. However, during most of this time the entire field, industry and professional alike, seems to have been bemused by the problem of nonphysiologic sources. Electrocautery, microwave ovens, electric shavers, and a whole host of exogenous electromagnetic interfering signals were recognized as potentially interfering with pacemaker function. This represented a challenge to the engineering-industrial community, which has been met well. Pacemakers were rapidly made substantially insensitive to the largely foreign signals of all the exogenous devices. That problem seems to be satisfactorily resolved.

While it is true that pacemakers produced in the last decade and one half are much less susceptible to EMI, they are not immune from many types found in the environment; particularly troublesome is the high-frequency current produced by electrosurgical and diathermy units, as well as EMI from cellular phones, communications equipment, and the industrial environment.

PACEMAKER MALFUNCTION DUE TO ELECTROSURGERY

Wajsczuk et al. (1969) reported a case in which a demand pacemaker in a patient was inhibited when the electrosurgical unit was activated during a transurethral resection procedure. They reported that although the cutting current inhibited the pacemaker, the coagulating current did not. A similar case was described by Smith and Wise (1971) in which both the cutting and coagulating current inhibited a demand pacemaker. They found that locating the dispersive electrode under the buttocks and relocating the wires carrying the electrosurgical current distant from the heart eliminated inhibition of the demand pacemaker.

Greene and Meredith (1972) pointed out that the newer demand pacemakers revert to fixed-rate pacing when interference is present. In transurethral resection operations on 12 patients they recommended the following precautions: (1) use a copious amount of conducting gel on the dispersive electrode; (2) place the dispersive electrode under the buttocks; (3) arrange the wires to the ESU so that they are perpendicular to the axis of the pacing lead in the heart, and (4) connect all equipment to the same ground. With these precautions, only one instance of pacemaker inhibition occurred when the ESU was activated.

Lerner (1973) reported another case of bipolar demand pacemaker inhibition in which the dispersive electrode was on the low thigh. During transurethral resection, cutting current inhibited the pacemaker, but coagulating current did not. In such cases, Lerner recommended activating the ESU using short bursts of current.

Inhibition of an implanted demand pacemaker by electrosurgical current was reported by O'Donoghue (1973), who wrote:

> Six months later (after pacemaker implantation), the patient underwent a transurethral resection of the prostate gland. The ground of the Bovie CSV is placed under the patient's buttock. As expected, continuous ECG monitoring was impossible during electrosurgery, because of the electrical interference. On two occasions following four to five seconds of electrocuting, the patient was noted to have tonic-clonic movements of the head and arms, and the carotid pulse could not be felt at this time. A magnet was placed over the pacemaker converting it into a fixed-rate unit, and no further episodes of inhibition occurred for the remainder of the operation. The patient had a good result, and no sequel from the temporary asystole.

O'Donoghue was aware of the need to direct the electrosurgical current away from the pacemaker and its leads when he wrote:

> Placing the indifferent electrode of the cautery under the buttocks of the patient should confine the current field to an area away from the pacemaker or endocardial electrodes, allowing electrosurgery to be carried out in safety, but as occurred in this patient, induction currents of sufficient magnitude to be picked up by the electrodes and inhibit the pacemaker can unfortunately still be generated.

In appraising the foregoing recommendations for placement of the dispersive electrode under the buttocks, it is useful to note that the surgical procedure was a transurethral resection and the buttocks location for the dispersive electrode directed the current away from the pacemaker. A better location for the dispersive electrode would be the thigh.

Domino and Smith (1983) elected to prevent electrosurgical inhibition of a demand pacemaker by placing a magnet on the chest to cause the pacemaker to operate in the fixed-rate mode. They reported:

A 59-year-old man with cervical spondylosis and a vocal cord lesion was scheduled for direct laryngoscopy and cervical laminectomy.

The patient had sick sinus syndrome "for which he had a permanent Medtronic Xyrel-VP right-ventricular, inhibited, unipolar, demand programmable pacemaker. Physical examination and preoperative laboratory studies were normal. An electrocardiogram revealed a paced rhythm at 70 beats/min.

…A toroidal ceramic magnet was then taped over the pacemaker to prevent interference from the cutting and coagulating current of the Birtcher electrocautery used during the laminectomy and a grounding pad was placed on a leg. The electrocautery was used sparingly for the first 45 min, during which time a spontaneous increase in heart rate to 100 beats/min with clear pacemaker artifact and ventricular capture was observed.

The pacemaker firing rate varied in multiples of ten (30, 70, 80, 90, 100), which corresponded to the possible programmable rate settings for this pacemaker.

From the foregoing it is clear that the pacemaker was variably affected by the electrosurgical current. Worthy of note is the fact that the active electrosurgical electrode was applied to the neck and the dispersive electrode was on a leg, placing the pacemaker lead directly in line with the electrosurgical current. Figure 13 illustrates this situation. Note that the pacing electrodes (P1, P2) are in line with the path taken by the electrosurgical current. The hazard is greater if a monopolar pacemaker is used because the spacing between the two electrodes is greater. Obviously, placing the dispersive electrode so that the electrosurgical current is directed away from the pacemaker lead is highly desirable.

Reprogramming of DDD pacemakers by electrosurgical current was reported by Bellott et al. (1984). In a study of 140 DDD pacer implants involving five different manufacturers, all pacemakers changed their mode of pacing to what is called the backup mode. All but one could be reprogrammed. They reported:

All pacemakers were implanted via the percutaneous sheath set, retained guide-wire technique. Electrosurgery was used to effect hemostasis. On occasion, because of skin-edge bleeding, electrosurgery was used with the pacemaker in the pocket. At no time was electrosurgery applied directly to the pacemaker. Units were in the pocket and a two-layer subcutaneous closure effected prior to application of electrosurgery to the skin edge. The site of the dispersive electrode was not given. As stated above, all units (except one) could be reprogrammed to the desired pacing mode. The unit that could not remained in the VVO mode.

A 1996 case investigated by the author provides another example of pacemaker malfunction due to electrosurgical current. A 75-year-old white male was taken to the operating room for surgery to relieve the pain of trigeminal neuralgia. He had an implanted cardiac pacemaker and had been pacemaker dependent since 1970 because of total A-V block. Full cardiorespiratory monitoring was employed during the procedure. The electrosurgical dispersive electrode was on the right thigh. When the active electrode of the ESU touched the skin of the back of the head, the patient became pulseless due to pacemaker failure. The patient was resuscitated with CPR and the application of a temporary cardiac pacer. The surgical procedure was abandoned and the patient was transferred to the ICU. Later, a DDD pacemaker was

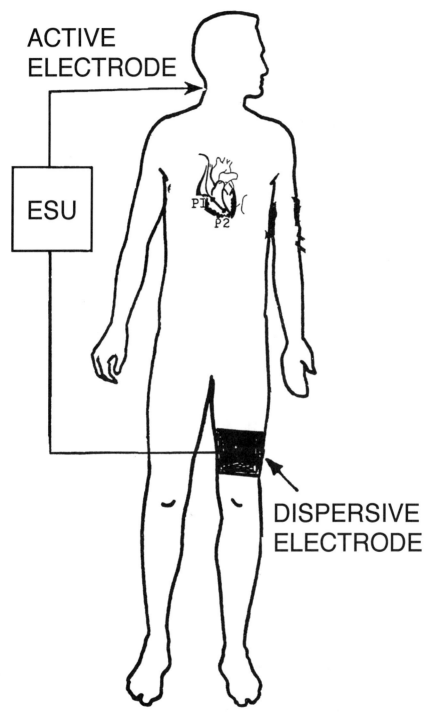

FIGURE 13 Pacing electrodes (P1, P2) in the heart and electrosurgical current applied to the neck via the active electrode with the dispersive electrode on the thigh.

implanted and the original (failed) pacemaker was not explanted. Radiographic evidence later revealed two implanted pacemakers. The patient recovered and the subsequent medical history will not be recounted.

In the foregoing case, the active electrode was applied to the back of the neck and the dispersive electrode was on the right thigh, placing the pacemaker lead directly in the path of the electrosurgical current, and the pacemaker was damaged irreversibly. This situation is that shown in Figure 13. If the dispersive electrode had been located to minimize the amount of electrosurgical current entering the pacemaker, it may well not have been destroyed. By placing the dispersive electrode over the left shoulder, the electrosurgical current would have been directed away from the pacemaker lead; in this case, the direction of current flow would be almost perpendicular to the axis of the pacemaker–catheter electrode axis.

ABANDONED PACEMAKER LEAD

An abandoned pacemaker lead is one that is not connected to a pacemaker, usually due to lead breakage. Very frequently the lead is not removed because of extensive fibrous tissue that anchors it. Usually the lead is cut off and a second pacing lead and pacemaker are implanted. Such an event is often discovered radiographically much later. Under some circumstances (e.g., the use of electrosurgery), this abandoned lead can induce serious cardiac arrhythmias, as the following example demonstrates.

Aggarwal et al. (1996) reported a case of ventricular fibrillation associated with a broken pacemaker lead and implantation of a new pacemaker. The patient, a 22-year-old male, had the original DDD pacemaker implanted because of sick sinus syndrome. The leads of this pacemaker were broken and abandoned because of extensive fibrosis. Aggarwal et al. stated:

> Two epicardial screw-in leads (Model 6917-53T, Medtronic) were placed on the inferior surface of the right ventricle via a subcostal approach. Threshold data for the replacement leads were 1.6 V, 3.1 mA with an R-wave of 7–8 mV and an impedance of 930 ohms. These leads were connected to a new VVI generator (Model 1204 META11, Telectronics). The pacemaker settings consisted of a pulse amplitude of 3.7 V, a pulse width of 375 µsec, a rate of 50 beats/min, a sensitivity of 2 mV, and a refractory period of 300 msec. The generator was replaced in the abdominal pocket of the old generator, and unipolar electrosurgery (Force 2, Valleylab) was used to provide hemostasis. A disposable, pre-gelled dispersal pad was placed on the patient's left anterior thigh. The electrosurgery unit (ESU) was used in a blend mode with cutting set at 20 and coagulation set at 30. The ESU had a return electrical monitoring system with an audible alarm for fault.
>
> During the use of the ESU, cardiac rhythm suddenly changed to ventricular fibrillation.
>
> Defibrillation was accomplished with external paddles at 300 joules, and a rhythm of ventricular tachycardia was then established. Ventricular tachycardia subsequently converted to sinus tachycardia following intravenous administration of a bolus of lidocaine (1.5 mg/kg). Heart rate subsequently decreased to 85 beats/min.

They explained this incident by stating:

> In the present case, we suggest that ventricular fibrillation occurred because of the direct conduction of current from the tip of the electrosurgery applicator to the surrounding tissues, and then via the exposed ends of the inner portion of severed pacing wires to the myocardium.

In the early days of cardiac pacing, the occurrence of ventricular fibrillation associated with electrosurgery and pacemaker leads was quite well known. For example, Titel and El Etr. (1968) reported an incident at a time when pacing electrodes were sutured directly to the myocardium. Then it was customary to first use a battery-operated external pacemaker before implanting a permanent pacemaker. They wrote:

> Electrodes were implanted in the myocardium and connected to an (external) pacemaker power pack by extension wires and alligator clamps. The clamp of one electrode was inadvertently placed on a wet drape near the incision. A Bovie electrocautery was used to achieve hemostasis prior to closure; the ground plate was under the patient's buttock. Each time the electrocautery was used the heart was observed to fibrillate. The artificially-paced rhythm resumed immediately each time cautery was discontinued. An alligator clamp noted to be touching the wet drapes was moved, contact with the drapes thus broken, and cautery continued without the recurrence of fibrillation. The patient required artificial pacing for about 6 h postoperatively after which the rhythm returned to normal. He recovered without further difficulty.

It should be noted that it is more likely that ventricular tachycardia, rather than fibrillation, was produced because true ventricular fibrillation rarely ceases by itself in man. However, ventricular tachycardia is a dangerous rhythm.

MOBILE TELEPHONE -GENERATED EMI

The possibility that mobile telephones may interfere with the operation of DDD pacemakers was investigated by Nowak et al. (1996). The authors studied 31 consecutive patients, 14 female, age range 61 ± 18 years, with high degree A-V block and a single-lead VDD pacemaker. Twelve patients had a Unity 292-07 (Intermedics), ten with a Thera 8949/8961 (Medtronic) and nine with a Sahir 600 (Vitatron) VDD pacemaker. After a complete pacemaker check the atrial and ventricular channels were programmed to minimum sensitivity thresholds (A: 0.1 = 0, 25 mV; V: 1.0 mV) and to unipolar ventricular sensing to simulate worst-case conditions. During continuous ECG recording, the antenna of a mobile phone (Orbitel 902.2 W, digital D-net) was brought in direct contact with the patient's skin, parallel to the pacemaker lead. Then the following operations were performed: connection to the net, making a call, ringing phase, receiving a call, and leaving the net. Thereafter, the pacemaker was interrogated and checked for any change of the programmed parameters. They concluded that in this group of patients with VDD pacemakers, no case of interaction was observed with the mobile phone. Although tested at minimum sensitivity thresholds with direct skin contact of the antenna, the single-lead VDD pacemakers examined were free from interference with a 2-W mobile phone in the digital D-net.

PACEMAKER MALFUNCTION DUE TO CELLULAR PHONES

Naegeli and Burkart (1996) investigated the effect of three hand-held and one transportable digital cellular telephones (GSM) on implanted cardiac pacemakers in 39 patients using the following pacemakers: 14 dual-chamber [DDD], 8 atrial-synchronized, ventricular-inhibited [VDD(R)], 17 ventricular-inhibited [VVI(R)], and four mobile phones with different levels of power output (2 and 8 W) in the standby, dialing, and operating modes. During continuous electrocardiographic monitoring, 672 tests were performed in each mode with the phones positioned over the implanted pacemaker and over the atrial and the ventricular electrode tip. The tests were carried out at different pacemaker sensitivity settings and, where possible, in the unipolar and bipolar pacing modes.

Each patient was tested with each type of mobile phone at maximal power output. In each operating mode, first the antenna and then the body of the mobile phones were placed (1) directly over the implanted pacemaker, (2) over the atrial electrode tip, (3) over the ventricular electrode tip; then they were moved slowly over the whole chest to detect possible interference with the pacemaker. Direct contact with the skin was avoided.

For each test series, the pacemakers were set to both the nominal and the maximal sensitivity settings. In a subset of 14 patients with VVI(R) pacemakers with programmable lead polarity, the whole test series was carried out in both the bipolar and unipolar pacing modes. All VVI(R) pacemakers were additionally tested in the rate-adaptive (R) mode with the nominal and most sensitive sensor settings. To avoid possible pacemaker inhibition due to myopotentials, the patients were asked to hold the phone with the hand opposite to the pacemaker implantation site. Each time that noise sensing was documented, the patient was asked to repeat the test without a phone to rule out myopotentials as the source of sensing. Then the test was repeated with the investigator holding the phone in the same position to prove reproducibility of the test result. Only reproducible results were considered to be due to electromagnetic interference.

The results of this carefully controlled study with digital communications (GSM) equipment revealed that in 7 (18%) of 39 patients, a reproducible interference was induced during 26 (3.9%) of 672 tests with the operating phones in close proximity (<10 cm) to the pacemaker. In 22 dual-chamber (14 DDD, 8 VDD) pacemakers, atrial triggering occurred in 7 (2.8%) of 248 and ventricular inhibition in 5 (2.8%) of 176 tests. In 17 VVI(R) systems, pacemaker inhibition was induced in 14 (5.6%) of 248 tests. Interference was more likely to occur at high power output of the phone and at maximal pacemaker sensitivity (maximal vs. nominal sensitivity, 6 vs. 1.8% positive test results, $p = 0.0009$). When the bipolar and unipolar pacing modes were compared in the same patients, ventricular inhibition was induced only in the unipolar mode (12.5% positive-test results, $p = 0.0003$).

The authors concluded that digital mobile phones in close proximity to implanted pacemakers may cause intermittent pacemaker dysfunction with inappropriate ventricular tracking and potentially dangerous pacemaker inhibition. Further, they recommended that:

> Pacemaker-dependent patients should be tested by their physicians for possible interferences before they use digital mobile phones. Furthermore, to minimize the risk of potentially dangerous pacemaker inhibition, their patients should be advised to hold the phone opposite to the site of implantation and not to carry it in a breast pocket close to the generator.

The testing referred to above involves recording the ECG with the telephone in the standby, dialing, receiving, and off modes.

In a similar multicenter study, the pacemaker response to cellular phones was determined in 980 patients using four types of digital and one type of analog cellular telephone. The ECG was monitored on all patients. Hayes et al. (1997) reported:

> The incidence of any type of interference was 20% in the 5533 tests, and the incidence of symptoms was 7.2%. The incidence of clinically significant interference was 6.6%. There was no clinically significant interference when the telephone was placed in the normal position over the ear. Interference was more frequent with single-chamber pacemakers (6.8%, P = 0.001) and more frequent with pacemakers without feed-through filters (28.9 to 55.8%) than with those with such filters (0.4 to 0.8%, P = 0.01).

They concluded:

> Cellular telephones can interfere with the function of implanted cardiac pacemakers. However, when telephones are placed over the ear, the normal position, this interference does not pose a health risk.

They added:

> Placement of the telephone over the pacemaker should be avoided. While the telephone is on, it should not be carried in a pocket over or close to the pacemaker.

PACEMAKER MALFUNCTION DUE TO MAGNETIC RESONANCE IMAGERS

In magnetic resonance imaging (MRI) there are three electromagnetic fields: (1) a high-intensity static field (1.5 T), (2) a high-frequency (64 MHz) field, and (3) gradient-coil fields (kilohertz). All of these fields are capable of interfering with the operation of cardiac pacemakers. Pacemaker manufacturers advise against placing patients with implanted pacemakers in MRI devices.

A study was carried out by Erlebacher et al. (1986) to investigate the type of pacemaker malfunction that resulted from exposing several different pacemakers to MRI fields. They studied four different DDD pacemakers (Cordis 233F, Intermedic 283-01, Medtronic 7000A, and Pacesetter 283) in a saline phantom under several conditions and with various imaging fields. Pacemaker output was monitored using electrocardiographic telemetry. All units paced normally with only the static magnetic field present. During imaging, all units malfunctioned, with total inhibition of atrial and ventricular output in three of the pacemakers. In the fourth, ventricular backup pacing was activated at high radiofrequency pulse repetition rates. However, the MRI scanner could trigger atrial output in this pacemaker at rates of up to 800/min. All malfunctions were a result of radiofrequency interference, whereas gradient and static magnetic fields had no effect. Despite magnetic field strengths adequate to close pacemaker reed switches, radiofrequency interference during MRI may cause total inhibition of atrial and ventricular output in DDD pacemakers, and can also cause dangerous atrial pacing at high rates. They concluded that MRI should be avoided in patients with these DDD pacemakers.

PACEMAKER MALFUNCTION DUE TO MICROWAVE -OVEN EMI

Rustan et al. (1973) investigated the 2450-MHz power density levels required to cause pacemakers to malfunction. The study involved nine dogs with implanted pacemakers and ten unimplanted pacemakers exposed to power density levels ranging from 1 to 10,000 μW/cm^2 . Demand and P-wave-triggered pacemakers were used; Table 12 identifies the types, many of which are no longer available. To simulate the emission from microwave ovens, a double modulation method was used. The main modulation was either 120 or 60 Hz; the second modulation ranged from 0.6 to 10 Hz. Each animal or unimplanted pacemaker was placed 370 cm from a pyramidal horn antenna that delivered the 2450-MHz electromagnetic energy. Electrocardiograms were obtained from the dogs and the frequency of the pulses from the unimplanted pacemakers was measured.

There was considerable variability in the responses of the various pacemakers, ranging from no effect at low power densities to reduced pacing rate, inhibition, and increased pacing rate. Figure 14 (A to I) presents the results for the implanted pacemakers and Figure 14 (J to S) presents the results for the unimplanted pacemakers. Two pacemakers (C and I) were inhibited at 8 μW/cm^2. Three unimplanted pacemakers (Q, R, S) were inhibited by 0.8 μW/cm^2. Rustan et al. stated that the maximum permissible level of radiation from microwave ovens is 5 mW/cm^2.

It is useful to note that this study was carried out in 1973 and some of these pacemakers are no longer in production. In addition, microwave ovens have improved, as have pacemakers. However, electromagnetic radiation from microwave ovens is still present and the degree to which it affects modern pacemakers is unclear. Hauser (1994) classifies microwave ovens as an unlikely source of pacemaker interference and microwave oven interference "has not been a concern for many years."

PACEMAKER MALFUNCTION DUE TO LOW-FREQUENCY EMI

In the earliest days of pacemaking, it was suspected that environmental signals could cause a ventricular pacemaker to malfunction. Calling attention to the paucity of literature on this subject, Carleton et al. (1964) tested a homemade pacemaker and a commercially available unit of the type that had been implanted in 26 patients.

TABLE 12
Pacemaker Types Exposed to Microwaves

A — Biotronik
B — Device Implanted 3821
C — Cordis Stanicor
D — Cordis Atricor
E — Vitatron
F — General Electric A2072D
G — American Optical 281013
H — Medtronic 5943
I — Medtronic 5842
J — Cordis Stanicor
K — General Electric A2072D
L — American Optical 281013
M — American Optical 281003
N — Medtronic 5942
O — Medtronic 5942
P — Medtronic 5942
Q — Medtronic 5842
R — Medtronic 5842
S — Medtronic 5842

Testing in the laboratory consisted of monitoring the pacemaker output on an oscilloscope. Another test consisted of placing the pacemaker electrodes on the tongue to feel the stimuli. Field tests were made with the oscilloscope powered by a portable alternator used to drive the oscilloscope.

The environments and the manner in which the pacemakers were tested are interesting and clearly demonstrated the need for improved pacemaker designs. For example, they reported:

The distributor of a 6-volt automobile electrical system produced acceleration of the pacemaker rate when the pacemaker was brought to within 6 cm of the distributor. An increase in the rate up to 450 impulses per minute occurred when any of the pacemakers was moved to within 1 cm of the distributor. Upon their withdrawal from the distributor field, however, a difference was noted between the two types of pacemakers; the locally made type produced no impulse for seven to ten seconds, while the commercially available pacemaker promptly resumed the original rate. The distributor of a 12-volt automobile electrical system produced similar alterations in pacemaker performance. The ignition coils of both automobiles produced occasionally sporadic, premature impulses without a fixed acceleration of rate in either type of pacemaker.

The spark plugs on a gasoline-powered lawnmower and a gasoline-powered alternator were tested. The spark plug of each was shown to alter pacemaker activity when the spark plug-pacemaker separation was less than 8 cm. As demonstrated with the distributor, a progressive acceleration of pacemaker rate occurred as the pacemaker was brought closer. All three pacemakers responded similarly.

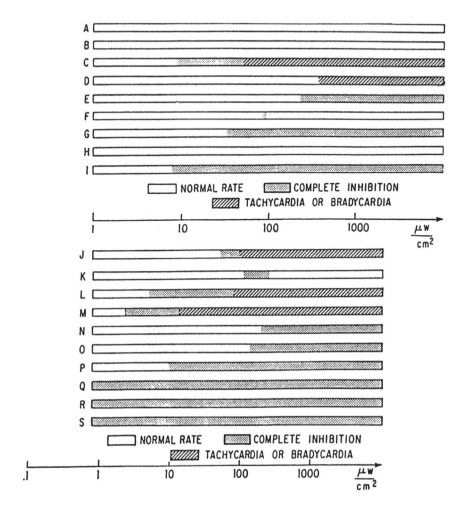

FIGURE 14 Responses of pacemakers (A–I) implanted in dogs and responses of unimplanted pacemakers (J–S) exposed to simulated microwave-oven energy. (Redrawn from Rustan, P.L., Hunt, W.D., and Mitchell, J.C. *Med. Instr.* 1973, 7: 185–188.

Carleton et al. (1964) identified 15 environmental items that did not affect the pacemakers. They even exposed their pacemakers to defibrillating current caused to flow through saline in which the pacemaker leads were immersed; transient arrest of pacing was encountered. With the highest defibrillator output, one pacemaker stopped permanently.

It is to be noted that these early pacemakers were not in a metal container; this issue was discussed as follows:

In most of these tests the pacemakers were covered only with three to four layers of towel wrapping. However, completely covering the pacemaker with the hands, thus interposing tissue of the approximate thickness of the usual subcutaneous pocket, did not protect against the effects of diathermy or automobile distributors.

The inherent electrical characteristics of oscillating circuits make them vulnerable to interference by electromagnetic activity in the environment. Since metals of high magnetic permeability, such as alloys with 80% nickel, have been used in other applications to provide electromagnetic shielding, a pacemaker was tested after its complete encasement in such an alloy. No protection from the effects of diathermy was observed, but the malfunction induced by automobile electrical parts was attenuated. With such shielding, the pacemaker output was stable at distances greater than 2 cm from distributors or spark plugs.

Modern pacemakers are in metal containers, only the leads protrude. Although the container affords shielding from much environmental EMI, high-frequency (electrosurgical and diathermy) radiofrequency current can still gain entry via the leads and cause pacemaker malfunction.

Several studies have been carried out in which pacemakers have been exposed to 50-, 60-, and 400-Hz fields. Some of these studies submerged the pacemakers in saline; others exposed patients with implanted pacemakers to these fields. In both cases, it was desired to determine the field strengths that would cause the pacemaker to malfunction. The following paragraphs summarize these studies.

A study designed to determine the susceptibility to electric and magnetic fields was reported by Jenkins and Woody (1978). Fifty-seven monopolar pacemakers, submerged in a non-conducting tank filled with 0.03M saline, were exposed to 50, 60, and 400 Hz electric fields. Twenty-six pacemakers, submersed in saline, were exposed to a 60-Hz magnetic field. In both cases the field strength could be increased until the pacemaker malfunctioned, as judged by oscilloscopic monitoring of the output pulses. In both cases, the voltage presented to the pacemaker electrodes was measured. The criteria for malfunction were (1) reversion from its normal mode of pacing to a fixed-rate mode, (2) inhibited, or (3) change of pacing rate beyond a range of 50 to 150/min. It was found that for directly injected interference (pacemaker in the saline tank), all of the pacemakers were susceptible to voltages ranging from 0.1 to 11.5 mV. The susceptibility for malfunction was greater for 50 to 60 Hz than for 400 Hz.

For the magnetically induced signal (pacemaker in saline tank surrounded by a Helmholtz coil), 30% malfunctioned when exposed to a field of 4 G. There was a nonlinear relationship between failure rate and magnetic field strength; about 4% failed when exposed to about 1.2 G.

When viewing the results of Jenkins and Woody (1978) it should be recognized that few, if any, of these early pacemakers are in patients today. Since then, pacemakers have been designed to reject such external signals. However, the test methods described by Jenkins and Woody are still applicable.

The effects of 50-Hz electric fields on implanted pacemakers was reported by Butros et al. (1983). The study involved 35 patients with 16 different types of pacemakers provided by six manufacturers. All were monopolar units and implanted in the pectoral region. Each patient stood between two electrodes that provided a uniform electric field, variable in intensity from 0 to 20 kV/m (rms). The current flowing through the subject was measured at each field strength and the pacemaker behavior was evaluated by the telemetered ECG.

As the field strength was increased, four types of response were noted: (1) normal sensing and pacing (i.e., no effect), (2) reversion to a fixed-rate mode, (3) slow and irregular pacing, and (4) slow and irregular pacing preceded by reversion to a fixed-rate mode. There were large differences among the different pacemakers for the field strengths required to produce these effects. Body current due to the electric fields in the range of 0 to 20 kV/m was measured because it is this current, flowing through the resistive tissues of the body, that develops a potential that enters the pacemaker via its electrodes. There was a linear relationship between body current and field strength. For a 172-cm subject, the body current was 200 μA (rms) for 20 kV/m. The body current for a taller subject was slightly higher and slightly less for a shorter subject. The body current required for reversion to a fixed-rate mode ranged from 37 to 200 μA. One pacemaker functioned normally at 200 μA of body current. The field strengths equivalent to these body currents are about 4 and 24 kV/m. Increasing the sensitivity of the pacemaker detection circuit lowered the field strength required for reversion. Commenting on their findings, Butros et al. (1983) concluded:

> The differences in behavior between different pacemaker models must be due to differences in the design of their sensing and filtration circuitry. It is encouraging that some models appear to be completely immune to interference by electric fields as high as 20 kV/m.
>
> Despite the abnormal behavior seen with some pacemaker models it should be stressed that power transmission lines, even those operating at the highest voltages (400 kV in the U.K.), should not be considered potentially hazardous to members of the general public who are fitted with pacemakers.

Butros et al. went on to state that the general public may be exposed rarely to in excess of 5 kV/m. It was observed from this study that all pacemakers tested (with the exception of two) needed more than 5 kV/m to change their behavior. They hastened to point out, however, that the electric field did not affect the programmability of the pacemakers, which functioned normally when the field was removed.

To determine the level of 50-Hz body current required to produce malfunction in implanted monopolar VVI pacemakers, Kaye et al. (1988) placed electrodes on the dorsal shoulders and on the feet of 18 patients and slowly increased the current. The pacemakers were manufactured by six different companies and the ECG was recorded during the trials. They reported that while increasing current:

> There was an initial period of normal pacemaker function followed by a variable period of mal-sensing, inappropriate pacing and intermittent complete inhibition. The duration of the period of inappropriate pacemaker behavior we have called the inappropriate window (I.W.) and have defined it as the difference between the minimum current producing inappropriate pacing and the minimum current producing reversion to fixed-rate pacing (interference mode). For all pacemakers the minimum current producing inappropriate pacing during bilateral current injection in the supine position occurred in the range 27–246 μA (median 88 μA). The width of the I.W. was in the range 2–90 μA, (median 15 μA). Further increase in the current produced reversion to interference or asynchronous mode in the range 29–255 μA (median 145 μA).

Kaye et al. (1988) also stated that posture and respiration were factors that determined the 50-Hz current for reversion. For example, there was a slight increase in the reversion current when the patient was in the sitting position. Deep inspiration reduced the current required for pacemaker reversion.

PACEMAKER MALFUNCTION DUE TO ARC-WELDING MACHINES

Using Siemens pacemakers with telemetered R-wave event markers to identify sensing, Marco et al. (1992) investigated the effect of several sources of environmental EMI on implanted pacemakers in 12 patients, and also *in vitro*. They reported that:

Electric arc-welding machines up to 225 A did not affect these pacemakers. Arc-welding machines using 1,000 A or more inhibited the *in vitro* test system within 1 or 2 meters of the weld or power generator. Electric welding machines with high-frequency voltage superimposed on the welding current affected the pacemaker when it was within 2 meters of the power unit and 1 meter of the weld. Very large industrial degaussing coils affected pacemakers within 2 meters. The test method using event records was found to be an effective addition to monitoring the pacemaker.

Marco et al. (1992) pointed out that there are several types of current used to deliver heat to the welding site; one type uses 50- or 60-Hz alternating current (AC), another uses direct current (DC), and another uses square waves. They also stated that high-frequency current may be added to AC or DC welding. Commenting on the propensity of arc welders to produce EMI, they stated:

AC welding using a square wave will probably result in significantly more EMI than one using sine wave since a square wave has many more frequency components. All the AC welding machines we tested used a sinusoidal waveform. Also, the high-frequency voltage that can be added to a DC or AC welding machine produced much more EMI than others. This was reflected in our results by more interference when these machines were used. Welders and welding engineers are generally aware of the high EMI from these types of welding machines.

An important factor recognized by Marco et al. (1992) was the way the cables to the welding machine were arranged; they stated:

Electric arc-welding machines up to 225 A without high frequency voltage and with the cables uncoiled were safe. If cables are coiled or if they are laid over the arm or shoulder of the person welding, the amount of EMI at the pacemaker will increase and it might be inhibited. Gas tungsten arc-welding machines and submerged arc-welding machines up to 1000 A were found to be safe for our patients to be in the vicinity, but not closer than approximately 1 meter to the weld. Many of these welding machines are automated at the weld site, so the operator might never need to be close enough to allow interference with their pacemaker.

AUTOMATIC IMPLANTED CARDIOVERTER DEFIBRILLATOR (AICD)

VENTRICULAR DEFIBRILLATION AND CARDIOVERSION

Because ventricular fibrillation (VF) has been associated with pacemaker and AICD function, and especially as a complication in electrosurgery, the nature of VF and the method of terminating it will be described briefly.

Ventricular fibrillation (VF) is a condition in which all of the muscle fibers of the ventricles, the main pumping chambers of the heart, contract and relax randomly and there is no cardiac output. Defibrillation is achieved by passing a high-intensity pulse of current through the ventricles via chest-surface electrodes. Patients with pacemakers are defibrillated and in this process the pacemaker can be damaged.

Figure 15A illustrates the ECG and blood pressure before the induction of VF (left) and during VF (beyond the arrow). Note the dramatic change in the ECG and the immediate fall in blood pressure. VF does not stop spontaneously in man and it is necessary to restore the circulation immediately by instituting cardiopulmonary resuscitation (CPR) and then defibrillating the ventricles. Typically, anterior-chest electrodes (D_1D_2), as shown in Figure 16, are used and a pulse of current (e.g., 40 to 50 amps, 5 to 10 msec) is passed through the adult thorax. Defibrillation is immediate, as shown in Figure 15B, and the heart usually starts to beat; if not, CPR is instituted until the heartbeat is restored or a higher energy shock is used to achieve defibrillation. Sometimes temporary pacing is needed.

Cardioversion is the term used when a pulse of current is delivered to chest electrodes to arrest atrial fibrillation; the term is also used when atrial tachycardia and ventricular tachycardia are treated. Giedwoyn (1971) reported a case in which a patient was implanted with a cardiac pacemaker and subsequently went into ventricular fibrillation. Five 400-J shocks were delivered with paddle electrodes and the pacemaker ceased to function.

When a patient with a pacemaker is defibrillated with anterior-chest electrodes (paddles), the pacing catheter electrodes (P1, P2, Figure 16) are virtually in line with the current flow between the defibrillating electrodes (D1, D2). Therefore, a substantial current can be delivered into the pacemaker via the pacing electrodes (P1, P2) and the pacemaker can be damaged.

A study of the amount of current entering a pacemaker due to defibrillating energy was reported by Lau et al. (1969). In his paper he stated that only one manufacturer (at that time) had placed protective circuitry (zener diodes) in the pacemaker. Since then pacemakers have been equipped with various types of protective circuitry. The amount of current entering the pacemaker will depend on the type of protective circuit, the intensity of the defibrillating current pulse, the location of the chest electrodes, and the location and spacing between the pacing electrodes (P1, P2). If the pacemaker lead is monopolar, i.e., one electrode on the catheter and the pacemaker case is the other electrode, the spacing between the electrodes is larger and the risk of pacemaker damage is greater. Although anterior-chest electrodes are used routinely for ventricular defibrillation, chest-to-back electrodes deliver current to the ventricles in a direction that is nearly at right angles to the

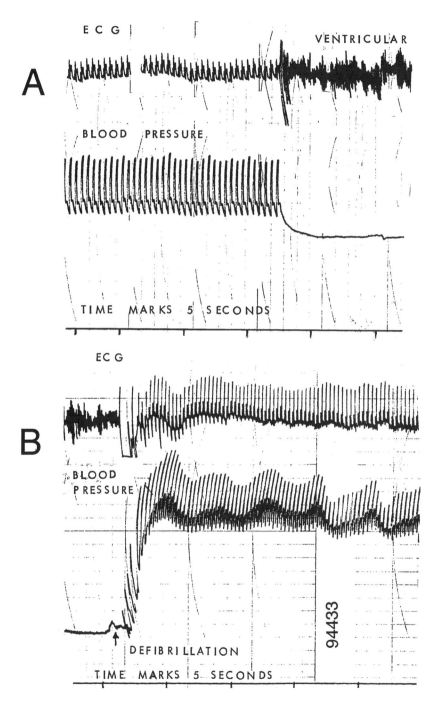

FIGURE 15 A The ECG and blood pressure before the induction of ventricular fibrillation (VF) (left of arrow) and during VF (right of arrow); (B) the delivery of a defibrillating shock and restoration of the ECG and blood pressure.

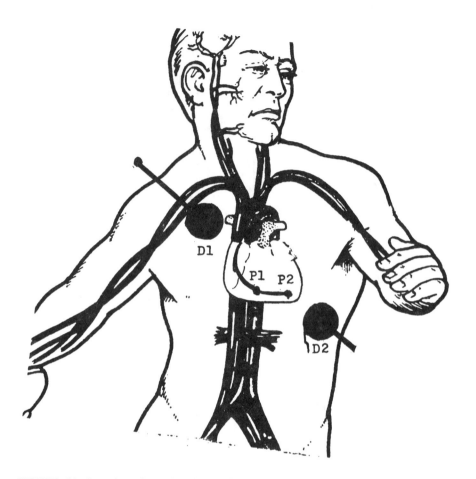

FIGURE 16 Location of anterior-chest defibrillating (paddle) electrodes (D1, D2) and a pacing catheter with electrodes (P1, P2) in the right ventricle.

axis of the pacing electrodes (P1, P2), and consequently much less current will enter the pacemaker via the pacing electrodes. Hauser (1994) made such a recommendation when he stated:

> The main concern during cardioversion and defibrillation (in a patient with a pacemaker) is the potential for circuitry damage. Also, energy may be coupled to the lead, causing myocardial damage. Another possible occurrence is inadvertent resetting of the pacemaker's programmed parameters.
>
> In order to minimize these possibilities, anterior–posterior paddles should be used rather than two anterior paddles. With anterior–posterior paddles, the energy is perpendicular to the plane of the lead and less energy is coupled to the lead. The paddles should be placed at least five inches from the pacemaker.

The myocardial damage referred to by Hauser results from high-current density at the interface between the pacing electrodes and myocardium due to the defibrillating current. The consequence of such damage is an increase in pacing threshold and loss of capture. When protective circuitry (Zener diodes and/or a low-loss capacitor) was placed in pacemakers in the early 1980s, the output impedance of pacemakers became low for the high-intensity defibrillating pulse of current; therefore, the current density at the pacing electrodes (P1, P2) becomes high during defibrillation and cardioversion. The price paid for pacemaker protection is temporary or permanent threshold increase and potential loss of capture. Levine et al. (1983) reported transient or permanent loss of capture in six pacemaker patients experiencing cardioversion or defibrillation.

Automatic implanted cardioverter defibrillators (AICDs) have been implanted in patients with an implanted pacemaker and malfunction resulted when the defibrillating shock was delivered. These cases are described in the section dealing with the AICD.

AUTOMATIC IMPLANTED CARDIOVERTER DEFIBRILLATOR OPERATION

The automatic implantable cardioverter defibrillator (AICD) is a device that detects a rapid ventricular rhythm and delivers a shock to terminate the arrhythmia. Originally devised by Mirowski et al. (1972), its first clinical feasibility was reported by Mirowski et al. in 1973. Now on the horizon is the automatic implantable atrial defibrillator, which is in preliminary clinical trials. Although effective, AICDs are not without complications, in the form of failure to deliver a shock, delivery of an inappropriate shock, complications following delivery of a shock, and susceptibility to EMI. The following paragraphs describe these complications, not all of which are device related.

Several different electrode systems, including catheter electrodes, transventricular patch electrodes, or a catheter electrode paired with a subcutaneous electrode, are used to detect the ventricular arrhythmia and to deliver the therapeutic shock. Sometimes a separate pair of electrodes is used to detect the electrogram.

Several different algorithms have been used to identify the type of ventricular arrhythmia (Jenkins and Caswell, 1996); however, at present, most are based on a rate criterion, the key requirement being detection of only the ventricular excitation waves. A few examples will be presented to illustrate the detection problem.

Figure 17A illustrates two normal ECG complexes, consisting of P, Q, R, S, and T waves. The P wave is produced by the atria; the Q, R, S, and T waves are produced by the ventricles. The three horizontal lines (1, 2, 3) identify three different sensing thresholds. Level 1 illustrates a threshold that detects only the R waves. Level 2 illustrates what is known as double counting, i.e., a threshold that detects both R and T waves, a situation that could cause the AICD to deliver an inappropriate shock if the R-wave rate is elevated. Level 3 illustrates gross oversensing in which the P, R, and T waves are sensed and the AICD is informed that the ventricular rate is three times the true rate, a condition that is very likely to result in delivery of an inappropriate shock to the ventricles. Obviously, single counting of the QRS wave is desirable to identify ventricular rate. The various waveforms that an AICD must distinguish will be described next.

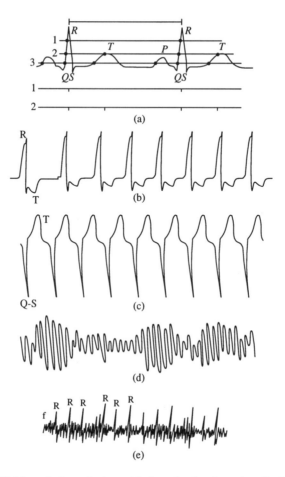

FIGURE 17 (A) Normal sinus rhythm with three levels of sensing (1, 2, 3); (B and C) ventricular tachycardia; (D) ventricular fibrillation; (E) atrial fibrillation.

Figures 17B and C illustrate ventricular tachycardia, a rapid ventricular rhythm that should be shocked; the shock strength required is less than that needed for defibrillation. Although Figures 17B and C both represent ventricular tachycardia, the focal origin of each is different.

Figure 17D illustrates ventricular fibrillation, a condition in which all cardiac pumping ceases and a defibrillating shock is mandatory. Note the high frequency and the waxing and waning of the amplitude of the fibrillation waves, making the detection task more difficult.

Figure 17E illustrates atrial fibrillation (f waves), a condition in which the ventricular (R-wave) rate is rapid and irregular. It is inappropriate for the AICD to deliver a shock to the ventricles because the arrhythmia is in the atria.

Despite the sensing difficulties just outlined, there is no doubt that for selected patients the AICD is a lifesaving device, with over 75,000 implants to date (Jenkins and Caswell, 1996). However, problems are beginning to appear in the form of failure to deliver a shock or delivery of an inappropriate shock. EMI can be implicated in these malfunctions. However, other complications exist which cannot be blamed on EMI; these will be dealt with later in this section.

AICD Control and Monitoring

Two-way communication is provided with an AICD via a telemetry link with the programmer that is placed on the skin above the implant which may be in the abdominal or pectoral region. The programmer can interrogate circuit function, e.g., sensing sensitivity and rate, energy setting and delivery, number of activations to date, etc. The programmer can also set certain operating parameters. In addition, an implanted AICD can be activated or deactivated by placing a small permanent magnet on the skin over the implant. Accidental deactivations are by no means unknown.

Effect of Electromagnetic Interference

Kim et al. (1987) reported the inadvertent delivery of shocks from an AICD in a patient with an implanted pacemaker. They stated:

> A patient with an automatic implantable cardioverter defibrillator (AICD) received two inadvertent shocks when a magnet was placed over the pacer during a routine permanent pacer check. Analysis of the rhythm strip suggested that both patient's QRS complexes (133 beats/minute) and asynchronous pacer artifacts (70 beats/minute) were counted by the AICD sensing system and exceeded the rate criteria of 153 beats/minute. This resulted in shocks from the AICD during sinus rhythm at 133 beats/minute. To avoid possible inadvertent shocks, an AICD should be deactivated while a magnet is placed over the pacemaker during a permanent pacer check.

During a routine follow-up, Bonnet et al. (1990) found five patients in whom the AICD was in the inactive state because of prior exposure to magnetic fields of various origins. They reported:

> Four of the five unsuspected deactivations clearly appeared to be from accidental contact with magnets in the everyday environment — two from magnetic bingo wands, one from a magnet placed in a jacket pocket next to the AICD, and one from a magnet inside a large stereo speaker which was carried by the patient. Once reactivated, interrogation revealed normally functioning devices without evidence of battery depletion. Fortunately, none of our patients had recurrent arrhythmias while their AICDs were inactivated. (The cause of the deactivation in the fifth patient was not identified.)

Another case of deactivation of an AICD by a loudspeaker was reported by Karson et al. (1989). The incident involved a patient who presented for a routine follow-up which revealed that the AICD had been deactivated. Karson et al. stated:

On careful questioning, however, he recalled that about 10 days earlier he had moved his large stereo speakers. In moving them, he had grasped the speaker cabinet from behind, put his arms around the unit, and lifted it up against his body. He remained in contact with the equipment for at least 30 seconds.

Checking with the manufacturer of the stereo speaker, we learned that the strength of the magnetic field at the speaker gap is rated at 1160 gauss. A hand-held gauss meter measured the magnetic strength in various places, with the probe in contact with the speaker cabinet: top, 6.1 gauss; bottom, 39.5 gauss; grill, 36 gauss; and baffle board, 48 gauss. Cardiac Pacemaker, the manufacturer of the cardioverter-defibrillator, indicated that a magnetic intensity of 10 gauss at the surface of the device is required for deactivation.

Another AICD deactivation due to the magnetic field of a loudspeaker was reported by Schmitt et al. (1991). The patient was a 60-year-old male who had a coronary artery bypass at which time an AICD was implanted. They reported:

> Since then, spontaneous discharges had not occurred. Upon follow-up in December, 1989, the device was deactivated and in standby function. A few days earlier, the patient had worked with a loudspeaker of his radio that came in close proximity to the AICD, thus deactivating the device. Positioning the loudspeaker approximately 20 cm in proximity to the AICD pocket reproducibly activated and deactivated the device. The magnetic field strength generated by the loudspeaker was 295 gauss at the surface, and 11 gauss at a distance of 5 cm. In October, 1990 the AICD was explanted and sent to the manufacturer for evaluation of possible reed switch problems. According to their information the activation/deactivation switch operated normally.

Another deactivation case was reported by Ferrick et al. (1991) which involved a 76-year-old lady bingo player who had an AICD implanted. Upon routine follow-up, the AICD was found to be deactivated and was promptly reactivated. She returned 2 months later for checkup and the AICD was again found to be deactivated. In pursuing the cause, Ferrick et al. (1991) stated:

> Only after an on-site review failed to detect a source of electromechanical interference did the patient's family allude to her routine of resting a "bingo wand" in her lap during weekly bingo tournaments. The wand was described as a small magnet encased in plastic that was designed to retrieve bingo chips. The recovered wand was shown to generate a magnetic field sufficient to activate and inactivate the AICD. With subsequent follow-up the AICD has remained in the active mode and has exhibited appropriate charge times. The patient no longer rests her bingo wand near the defibrillator while engaging in bingo competition.

Three cases of AICD malfunction due to EMI were reported by Schmitt et al. (1991). The first case was a 36-year-old male who experienced ventricular tachycardia and an AICD was implanted and functioned normally. Nine months later, a burst of ventricular tachycardia occurred which was not terminated by the AICD. Emergency transchest cardioversion was used to resuscitate the patient. Investigating this incident, Schmitt et al. reported:

One month prior to his last VT episode, the patient was in close contact with magnetized screws needed for construction of book shelves. These magnetized screws, when in close proximity to the implanted device for 30 seconds reproducibly deactivated the AICD. The strongest magnetic field generated by the magnetized screws was approximately 30 gauss. In 1989 the AICD was replaced because of battery depletion. The device was sent to the manufacturer. According to information of the manufacturer this AICD had a random component failure: one of the reeds of the reed switch was bent at an incorrect angle causing the AICD to be more sensitive to magnetic fields.

The second case reported by Schmitt et al. (1991) was a 66-year-old male with coronary heart disease and recurrent ventricular tachycardia. An antitachycardia pacemaker (with an externally inhibiting magnet) was implanted. Later, an AICD was implanted (August 1987). In a follow-up study Schmitt et al. (1991) reported:

At the first 1-month follow-up, the AICD was deactivated by the magnetic activator of the antitachycardiac pacemaker. This magnetic interference and disabling of the AICD occurred even at a distance of 40 cm. The patient had carried the activator in his pocket, thus deactivating the AICD. The magnetic field strength generated by the antitachycardia pacemaker magnetic activator was 630 gauss at the surface, and 2.4 gauss at 5 cm. The pacemaker was explanted and replaced by an automatic, anti-tachycardiac pacemaker (Intertach. Intermedics, Inc., Freeport, TX, USA).

Schmitt's third case involved AICD deactivation by the magnetic field of a loudspeaker. This case was described earlier in this section.

Discharge of an AICD by a hand-held radiofrequency remote controller for a toy car was reported by Ching Man et al. (1993). The patient was a 46-year-old male with a history of ischemic heart disease. A third-generation, multiprogrammable AICD was implanted. Ching Man et al. reported:

One year after implantation, the patient reported an episode of defibrillator discharge while operating a hand-held remote control to a radiofrequency modulated toy car (2-Channel Transmitter, Model #FP-2PBKA, Futaba Corporation of America, Irvine, CA, U.S.A., frequency 75.950 MHz, 12-volt battery source). The patient did not experience any symptoms prior to the defibrillator discharge. Investigation showed that: When the remote control was turned on and placed next to the pulse generator in the left upper quadrant of the abdomen, oversensing occurred. This oversensing was dependent on the distance between the remote control and the device, the orientation of the remote control in the frontal plane, and the length of the remote control antenna. Oversensing occurred only when the remote control was within 8 cm of the ICD. Interference was observed only when the antenna was angled between 60–120° in the frontal plane and when the antenna was extended >45 cm. Noise detection was eliminated when a ground wire was attached to the antenna and when the antenna was detached from the remote control. The various features of the remote control transmitter such as the steering and speed did not affect the level of signal interference. Finally, no signal interference was detected when an aluminum shield was placed between the pulse generator and the remote control.

Embil et al. (1993) investigated a case involving a 48-year-old male with dysplasia who received an AICD because of a drug-refractory arrhythmia. Following recovery the patient was anxious to return to work as an arc welder. The work site was evaluated for potential interference with the AICD and Embil et al. reported:

> Telemetered intracardiac electrograms (EGM) and marker pulses (MP) were recorded while the patient used the arc welder (Model 250-DC-CP-TS, Auckland Canada Ltd., Miller Electric Co., Appleton, WI, USA) and performed spot welding (Rex Welding and Engineering Company, Type F.P.U., Markum, Ontario, Canada), and also while he stood near a high voltage transformer (Model DT3, Westinghouse Electric Corp., Somerset, NJ, USA). The sensitivity of the ICD was maintained at its usual maximum setting of 0.3 mV. During the course of his work, his lower thorax (where the ICD was implanted) came within 10 cm of the cable supplying electricity to the arc welding electrode holder, and between 10–50 cm from the spot welding electrode.

During arc welding the ECG telemetered from the AICD showed infrequent spikes with an amplitude of about half of that of the QRS wave, but they were not sensed by the AICD. No false (R-wave) marker pulses were sensed. Magnetic field strengths were measured in the environment of the arc welder. Embil et al. (1993) reported:

> The arc welder was operated at settings at the upper end of the operational range (200 A and 30 V, welding 1/4 inch steel using a 0.035-mm wire electrode). At a distance of 10 cm from the electrical cable supplying the welding electrode, the magnetic fields measured were typically 1 gauss (G), maximum 3 G. The measured frequency of pulsing was 70 Hz. The high-frequency component created by the arc was extremely small at 1–3 mG.

They continued:

> Magnetic field in excess of 90 G will definitely close the reed switch of this device, but constant DC magnetic fields of 20 G or more may result in closure. Among the items of equipment at the patient's workplace, only the arc welding apparatus generated a DC magnetic field that, although pulsed rather than constant, could conceivably have caused the switch to close. Since the maximum DC field measured at a distance of 10 cm from the cable was only 3 G, its intensity was clearly insufficient to affect the reed switch.
>
> The measured field strengths at the patient's place of work were lower than expected. Levels of 3–10 G may be compared with the fields generated by such common household objects as electric shavers, microwave ovens, and hair dryers, which generate AC fields of up to 1.5, 2, and 20 G, respectively.

The decision in this case was that the patient could return to work as an arc welder. Nonetheless, the following caveat was offered:

> Nevertheless, the general ability of patients fitted with electronic devices to work in the presence of strong electromagnetic fields remains uncertain and our results are only directly applicable to patients fitted with an ICD who are exposed to these specific varieties of welding equipment kept in good repair.

The possibility that operating heavy industrial machinery (arc welders, 200-HP motors, and a locomotive starter) could interfere with an AICD was investigated by Fetter et al. (1996). The study involved 11 patients working about 1 ft from these devices, which draw substantial electric current and produce appreciable magnetic fields. In three of the patients the AICD was implanted pectorally, and in the remainder the implants were in the abdomen. The AICDs used bipolar sensing with the electrodes spaced 1 cm. The emitted electromagnetic energy spectrum was measured from 0.01 Hz to 100 MHz. The counters in all AICDs were interrogated by telemetry to identify malfunction.

The measured electromagnetic spectrum was almost uniform over the frequency range, with a slight peak at 2 MHz. Commenting on the effects on the AICDs, they stated:

> At no time was any ventricular tachycardia or ventricular fibrillation counteractivated by the radiated electromagnetic interference for any test conducted on any patient. There was no damage or reprogramming of any implanted defibrillator during the tests.

Mindful of the fact that the results were obtained with only 11 subjects and with only two types of AICD, Fetter et al. (1996) provided recommendations for others by stating:

> However, it would be prudent to provide an extra margin of safety before the patient returns to an electrically hostile work site by 1) having a technical consultant from the device manufacturer conduct a comprehensive electromagnetic interference test with patients at their site; 2) increasing the defibrillator sensitivity to 0.6 mV, programming the number of intervals to detect ventricular tachycardia to a minimum of 16, and programming the number of intervals to detect ventricular fibrillation to a minimum of 18; 3) determining the type of electrical equipment that the patient will be operating and assuring that appropriate electrical grounding is maintained in good condition; 4) ensuring that the patient's implantable defibrillator is 2 ft from the electrical source of the electromagnetic interference; 5) having patients wear gloves to avoid inadvertent contact with circuit electrical potentials; 6) advising patients to stop operating the electrical equipment if they experience a shock or lightheadedness and to immediately contact their primary physician.

AICD Malfunction Not Due to EMI

It is important to recognize that not all AICD malfunction is due to EMI. There are circumstances that cause an AICD to deliver an inappropriate shock or fail to deliver a shock. For example, Jenkins and Caswell (1996) reviewed the literature and stated that atrial tachycardia and atrial fibrillation, both of which drive the ventricles at a rapid rate, often cause an AICD to deliver an inappropriate shock. Figure 17E shows atrial fibrillation; note the rapid ventricular (R-wave) rate and the variability in the amplitude of the R waves. Because the arrhythmia resides in the atria, it is inappropriate to deliver a shock to the ventricles.

Pacemaker Patients and the AICD

It is not surprising that patients with implanted pacemakers receive an AICD and the opportunity for interaction is omnipresent. The pacemaker could be a ventricular-demand type or a DDD type, which can pace both the atria and ventricles or be triggered by atrial activity. Regardless of type, the pacemaker stimuli (spikes) are delivered to the heart and the AICD monitors the ventricular activity. Echt (1984) pointed out that an AICD can sense a ventricular pacing pulse and the evoked ventricular response, especially if the intraventricular conduction time is long; this is an example of double counting. Likewise, if the atria and the ventricles are paced by a DDD pacemaker, the AICD may sense the atrial pacing spike, the ventricular pacing spike, and the evoked ventricular response; this is an example of triple counting and could cause delivery of an inappropriate shock. The likelihood of sensing pacing pulses is greater with a monopolar pacing system.

A remarkable record of pacemaker-induced AICD inhibition in a patient in ventricular fibrillation was published by Kim et al. (1986). The patient was a 60-year-old lady who had a pacemaker implanted before AICD implantation. Kim et al. reported:

> The unipolar ventricular demand pacemaker implanted previously was not inhibited entirely during VF, presumably because of low amplitude of endocardial signals during VF. As a result, large unipolar pacer artifacts occurred randomly. The AICD failed to detect VF for more than 45 seconds, and external direct current defibrillation was required. The unipolar pacemaker was replaced by a bipolar pacemaker, with resolution of the problem. The sensing time (from the onset of arrhythmia to discharge of the AICD) was 22 seconds.

Cohen et al. (1988) investigated the interaction between both monopolar and bipolar implanted pacemakers and the AICD in nine patients. Studies were performed by inducing ventricular fibrillation and observing the AICD response. They reported:

> Undersensing of ventricular fibrillation by the permanent pacemakers caused inappropriate pacemaker stimuli, which caused undersensing of ventricular fibrillation by the AICD in three of four patients with unipolar pacemakers. After an AICD discharge, pacemaker noncapture was seen in eight of 22 episodes for an average 4.9 seconds and inability to sense was seen in 11 of 20 episodes for an average 9.0 seconds. Counting of pacemaker stimuli and QRS by the AICD caused inappropriate discharges.

Worthy of note in the foregoing is the fact that the postshock pacing threshold increased, as evidenced by the temporary loss of capture. This phenomenon occurs with closed-chest defibrillation of patients with implanted pacemakers. Cohen et al. recommended that only bipolar pacemakers should be used in patients with AICDs.

Similar experiences with AICDs implanted in 30 pacemaker patients were reported by Calkins et al. (1990), who wrote:

Seventeen percent of patients receiving an AICD at The Johns Hopkins Hospital also had a permanent pacemaker implanted before (16 patients), at the same time as (2 patients) or after (12 patients) AICD implantation. Four types of interactions were noted: (1) transient failure to sense or capture immediately after AICD discharge (seven patients); (2) oversensing of the pacemaker stimulus by the AICD, leading to double counting (one patient); (3) AICD failure to sense ventricular fibrillation resulting from pacemaker caused by AICD discharge (three patients).

Particularly interesting is their conclusion, which stated:

Pacemaker system malfunction occurs frequently after an AICD discharge but is a transient phenomenon and does not appear to have clinical consequences. Double counting of pacemaker stimuli or both pacemaker stimuli and the evoked depolarization is unusual and the failure of the AICD to sense ventricular fibrillation has not been observed with bipolar pacemakers set at standard outputs. A previously unreported interaction, pacemaker reprogramming to a backup mode by an AICD discharge, occurs with an unexpectedly high frequency and may have important consequences. Although many of these potential adverse interactions may occur and must be screened for before discharge to minimize their occurrence, clinically important interactions between the two devices appear to be uncommon.

Khastgir et al. (1991) reported death due to ventricular arrest in two patients with AICDs caused by A-V block following delivery of the AICD discharge. They stated that presently FDA-approved AICDs do not have a backup pacing modality and reported:

These cases illustrate the need for backup ventricular pacing and the ability to scan and retrieve the electrical events surrounding automatic implantable cardioverter-defibrillator discharges. Future technological advances addressing these issues will hopefully allow further decrease in sudden cardiac death incidence and enhance applicability to these high risk patients.

From the foregoing it is clear that there are many possible types of interaction between an AICD and an implanted pacemaker. Failure to sense ventricular fibrillation because of counting pacemaker spikes can prevent an AICD from delivering a shock. Counting pacemaker spikes and evoked ventricular responses can cause delivery of an inappropriate shock. Likewise, the rapid ventricular rate in atrial tachycardia, flutter, or fibrillation can cause an AICD to deliver an inappropriate shock to the ventricles. The increase in pacing threshold following a defibrillator shock is not uncommon and results in loss of capture. Moreover, A-V block often follows a defibrillating shock and emphasizes the need for backup pacing. Finally, the issue of an AICD shock reprogramming a pacemaker is a hazard that needs to be investigated.

It is clear that if an implanted AICD is to be used in a patient with a pacemaker, the preference is for a bipolar system. However, more important for the future is an AICD that contains a pacemaker so that the two devices can communicate with each other. Despite the future appearance of such a dual-function device, Spotnitz et al. (1992) cautioned:

> Even when dual-function devices become available, special situations will arise that require familiarity with the techniques described. Detection of pacemaker spikes by the ICD can lead to either inappropriate ICD discharges or failure of the ICD to detect and fire in ventricular fibrillation. These problems can be avoided by use of bipolar pacemakers and lead configurations physically separating the lead systems.

ELECTROSTATIC DISCHARGE

INTRODUCTION

Electrostatic discharge (ESD) pertains to the transfer of electric charge from a body at one potential to a body at a different potential. The most familiar example is the charge that is accumulated on a subject after walking on a carpet in a dry room and a spark discharge occurs when another person or object is touched. Other examples are the sparks drawn when combing the hair or removing clothing made of synthetic fabric. Although the voltages can be high, the discharge lasts only microseconds. Dash and Straus (1995) stated that the capacitance of a standing subject is typically 150 pF. Parenthetically, the dielectric breakdown (arcing voltage) for dry air is about 25,000 V/cm for a point source. The breakdown is slightly higher for spherical bodies. It is to be noted that the relative humidity is an important factor in ESD; a low relative humidity favors the genesis of electrostatic charge buildup.

ESD TESTING

In the U.S., professional groups are developing procedures for ESD testing. However, in Europe, there is a protocol for testing the susceptibility of devices to ESD; it is contained in the International Electrotechnical Commission document 1000-4-2 (1995). Briefly, the method exposes the device under test to a graded high-voltage discharge to determine the voltage for malfunction. The method employs a capacitor (150 pF) connected to a ground plane (grounded metal sheet) on which the device rests. The other (positive) side of the capacitor is connected to a resistor (330 ohms), which is connected to a spherical electrode at the tip of a wand. The test starts with 2 kV on the capacitor. As the charged sphere is brought toward the device the intervening air becomes ionized and a current starts to flow and evidence of device malfunction is sought. The test is repeated ten times at each selected site on the device under test. The procedure is repeated by incrementing the voltage in 2-kV steps until 8 kV is reached. The voltage for device malfunction is identified.

Three modes of testing are employed: (1) the charged sphere on the wand is brought toward the ground plane on which the device rests, (2) the charged sphere is advanced toward the chassis of the device, and (3) the charged sphere is advanced toward connector shells, displays, keyboards, switches, etc. on the device. During these three modes of testing, the lowest voltage for malfunction is identified. Ideally, malfunction should not occur at 8 kV.

Mechanism of Action

ESD can affect medical devices in many ways, ranging from a transient event to permanent malfunction. Because many medical devices contain electronic circuitry with solid-state components (analog and digital), ESD can reveal itself in bizarre ways. Proving that ESD was the cause of a malfunction is not always easy because an on-site test for reproducibility is not always possible. However, witnessing an arc in association with a device malfunction confirms the diagnosis of ESD as the culprit.

When no arc is witnessed it is difficult to establish that the malfunction or failure is due to ESD. However, the static discharge produced when a subject is touched while a bioelectric event is being recorded can produce a spike in the recording; such an event is reproducible. Of course, a higher intensity ESD can enter an amplifier input via a disconnected electrode lead and damage the input stage, rendering the amplifier permanently inoperative unless protective circuitry has been provided. The same type of fault can occur with both electrodes connected to the patient. In this case the discharge follows the common-mode path.

ESDs of even moderate intensity can reprogram a microprocessor that may be controlling a ventilator, drug-infusion pump, a wheelchair, etc., resulting in disastrous consequences. In some cases, it may only be necessary to reprogram the microprocessor.

ESD Incidents

The most complete listing of ESD incidents can be found in a paper by Silberberg (1993), who reported the following items: (1) the loose-lead alarm failed to sound and the respiration sensitivity was reduced in apnea monitors due to component damage from ESD; (2) the respiratory or heart-rate alarms of apnea monitors failed to sound due to electrostatic discharges to the screws on the setting knobs; (3) electrostatic interference influenced the normal operation of the synchronization unit of a ventilator in a hospital in Europe. Customers were informed not to use the synchronization until ESD caused "system check" alarms or failure of an infusion pump; (4) ventilators stopped cycling while on patients in a hospital. The ventilators were found to be susceptible to ESD; (5) ESD caused CMOS components to latch up, disabling apnea monitors without an alarm until power was turned first off and then on; (6) ESD caused unintended movement of a gamma camera, which could potentially cause a patient to be crushed; (7) ESD caused infusion pumps to shut down, sometimes without activating an alarm; (8) in radiation therapy devices, ESD caused the source to turn on, the display to blank, unintended gantry movement, or timer failures which resulted in possible patient overdose. Recovery required first switching the device off. In one instance a discharge from an operator to the timer of a radiation therapy system caused the timer's display to blank just as the treatment had begun. The treatment was terminated by opening the treatment room door; (9) ESD from an operator to the membrane switch of an internal feeding pump resulted in continuous alarm and destructive failure of the firmware EPROM; and (10) ESD affected infant radiant warmers, causing the heater to turn on or off, alarm failure, and the display to become blank or corrupted.

An unusual incident of roller-pump failure in a heart-lung machine was reported by Leahy et al. (1993). During an operation, the pump indicator signaled a failure. The pump was restarted and the machine was checked and functioned normally. Several weeks later, multiple failures occurred with the same and other machines. It was found that an electrostatic discharge near the machine could stop the pump.

During the operation, the perfusionist made notes on a plastic-backed clipboard. Leahy et al. stated:

> When the clipboard was placed on the front of the pump module, its electrostatic charge was released onto the pump case, causing the pump to fail.

Pursuing the matter further, Leahy et al. reported:

> The clipboard is made of plastic with a metal clip. When it was rubbed against the operating room uniform, it built up and stored an electrical charge.

They continued:

> At our institution, preventive measures have been adopted to reduce the incidence of pump failure from static discharge. These include discontinuing the practice of placing the clipboard on the pump module and maintaining the relative humidity at the required levels.

A good example of susceptibility to ESD was reported by Martin (1993), who tested a laboratory blood sampler having an LCD display. He stated:

> The product consisted of a totally plastic case with conductive coating applied on the interior surfaces. A tongue-and-groove joint was used to affix the front and back half of the seams of the chassis. The failures experienced included resets of the processor or initiation of unexpected mechanical movements.

Careful examination of the device revealed that inadequate contact existed between the conductive coatings on the front and back of the device. This lack of contact caused a high field to exist at the seam where discharges occurred. In addition, there was inadequate grounding of the circuit card and LCD frame to the chassis. When these improvements were made, Martin stated that the device was immune to the 8-kV test specified by IEC 801-2 (now 1000-4-2).

EFFECT OF ESD ON HUMAN SUBJECTS

Everyone has perceived an ESD as a mild, often surprising shock. The issue of whether such a shock can do harm is less well known. McCarty and Glasser (1977) noted that an ad hoc commission stated that static electric discharges could induce fatal cardiac arrhythmias. Because of this it was recommended that carpet not be placed in critical care areas. After searching the literature, McCarty and Glasser could find no basis for this recommendation and initiated a dog study to evaluate this hazard.

Using seven anesthetized dogs, they placed a #5 bipolar pacing catheter in the right ventricle and confirmed its proximity to the endocardium by recording the cardiac electrogram and testing the pacing threshold. Static-electricity discharges were generated "by shuffling our shod feet over synthetic or wool carpet. Static charges were discharged from the fingertips and measured through a 50.1-megohm resistor into a Tektronix storage scope. More than one spike, i.e., double static discharge, was induced occasionally by incomplete initial contact with the catheter tip. Similar static charges were then applied directly on the external end of the pacemaker wire leading in the distal electrode within the right ventricle."

They reported:

> The voltage of static charges reached 22,000 volts. The charges varied with the shoes worn, type of rug, duration of shuffling, and the day — presumably related to temperature, humidity, etc. The perceptible level of shock to the finger was established at two to three thousand volts. The energy delivered, as measured through the 50.1-megohm resistor, was calculated at 4.3 millijoules (4300 microjoules) for an 8,000 volt discharge.

They continued:

> Static discharges exceeding 2,000 volts uniformly resulted in paced beats, unless delivered in the absolute refractory period. Ventricular beats were often initiated by discharges below the level of perceptible shock. In fact, a single gliding movement of one's foot across the rug generated a sufficient charge to pace the heart. This allowed repetitive pacing at rates nearing 60/min. Powerful shocks delivered in the vulnerable period of the cardiac cycle did not produce repetitive tachyarrhythmias.

Although ventricular fibrillation was not produced in normal dog hearts, the creation of myocardial infarction by coronary ligation (three dogs) allowed the induction of ventricular fibrillation. They reported on one dog:

> A discharge approximating 6,000 volts clearly initiated ventricular fibrillation. This appears to have resulted from a double discharge in which current was repetitively delivered after the initial discharge had produced a ventricular premature beat (VPB). This secondary shock occurred within the vulnerable period of the VPB and initiated VF, electrical countershock returned the rhythm to sinus.

McCarty and Glasser emphasized that a single shuffle of one foot provided enough ESD to evoke a ventricular beat. They stated that the type of shoe was an important factor; those that produced measurable friction generated enough ESD. Shoe coverings, such as booties used in operating rooms, are not effective generators of static electricity.

REFERENCES

AAMI Association for the Advancement of Medical Instrumentation. 3330 Washington Blvd., Arlington, VA 22201-4598.

Aggarwal, A., Farber, N.E., Kotter, G.S., et al. Electrosurgery-induced fibrillation during pacemaker replacement. *J. Clin. Mon.* 1996, 12: 339–342.

Bassen, H.I., Ruggera, P.S., Casamento, J. Changes in susceptibility of a medical device resulting from connection to full-size model of a human. Proc. 14th Annual Int. Conf. of the IEEE Engineering in Medicine and Biology Society, 1992. pp. 2832–2833.

Bellott, P.H., Snads, S., and Warren, J. Resetting of DDD pacemakers due to EMI. *PACE* 1984, 7: 169–172.

Birnbaum, M.R. and Stasz, P. Apnea monitoring system. U.S. Patent 4,580,575, April 8, 1986.

Bonnet, C.A., Elson, J.J., Fogoros, R.N., et al. Accidental deactivation of the automatic implantable cardioverter defibrillator. PACE 1990, 13: 546.

Bostrom, U. Interference from mobile telephones. *Newsl. Clin. Eng. Div. IFMBE* 1991, 10 (November).

Bren, S.P.A. Revealing the RF safety issue in cellular telephones. *IEEE Eng. Med. Biol.* 1996, May–June.

Butros, G.S., Mate, J.C., Webber, R.S., et al. The effect of power frequency high intensity electric fields on implanted cardiac pacemakers. *PACE* 1983, 6: 1282–1291.

Calkins, H., Brinker, J., and Veltri, E.P. Clinical interactions between pacemakers and automatic implanted cardioverter defibrillators. *J. Am. Coll. Cardiol.* 1990, 16(3): 666–673.

Canadian Standard Association, 235 Montreal Road, Ottawa, Ontario, Canada. Code for the Use of Flammable Anesthetics and Canadian Standard (22.2).

Carleton, R.A., Sessions, R.W., and Graettinger, J.S. Environmental influence on implantable cardiac pacemakers. *J.A.M.A.* 1964, 190: 160–162.

Ching Man, K., Davidson, T., Langberg, J.J., et al. Interference from a hand-held radiofrequency remote control causing discharge of an implantable defibrillator. *PACE* 1993, 16: 1756–1758.

Clifford, K.J., Joyner, K.H., Stroud, D.B., et al. Mobile telephones interfere with medical electrical equipment. *Austral. Phys. Eng. Sci. Med.* 1994, 17(1): 23–27.

Cohen, A.L., Wish, M.H., Fletcher, R.D., et al. The use and interaction of permanent pacemakers and the automatic implantable cardioverter defibrillator. *PACE* 1988, 11: 704–711.

Dash, G. and Straus, I. Testing for ESD immunity. *Compliance Eng.* 1995, B5–B11.

Domino, K. and Smith, T.C. Electrocautery-induced reprogramming of a pacemaker using a precordial magnet. *Anesth. Analg.* 1983, 62: 609–612.

Echt, D.S. Potential hazards of implanted devices for the electrical control of tachyarrhythmias. *PACE* 1984, 7: 580–587.

Embil, J.M., Geddes, J.S., Foster, D., et al. Return to arc welding following defibrillator implantation. *PACE* 1993, 16: 2313–2316.

Erlebacher, J.A., Cahill, P.T., Pannizzo, F., et al. Effect of magnetic resonance imaging on DDD pacemakers. *Am. J. Cardiol.* 1986, 57: 437–440.

Ferrick, K.J., Johnston, D., Kim, S.G., et al. Inadvertent AICD inactivation while playing bingo. *Am. Heart J.* 1991, 121: 206–207.

Fetter, J.G., Benditt, D.G., Stanton, M.S., et al. Electromagnetic interference from welding and motors on implantable cardioverter-defibrillators tested in the electrically hostile work site. *J. Am. Coll. Cardiol.* 1996, 28(2): 423–427.

Foster, K. Interference from cellular phones. *Sci. Eng. Biomed.* 1994, December.

Furman, S. Electromagnetic interference. *PACE* 1982, 1–3.

Geddes, L.A. Technical note: observations of intermittent electromagnetic interference on impedance respiration monitors. *J. Clin. Eng.* 1995, 20(2): 151–155.

Geddes, L.A., Hoff, H.E., Hickman, D.M., and Moore, A.G. The impedance pneumograph. *Aerospace Med.* 1962, 33: 28–33.

Geddes, L.A., Hoff, H.E., Hickman, D.M., et al. Recording respiration and the electrocardiogram with common electrodes. *Aerospace Med.* 1962, 33: 791–793.

Geddes, L.A. and Valentinuzzi, M.E. Temporal changes in electrode impedance while recording the electrocardiogram with dry electrodes. *Ann. Biomed. Eng.* 1973, 1(3): 356–367.

Giedwoyn, J.O. Pacemaker failure following external defibrillation. *Circulation* 1971, 44: 293.

Greene, L.F. and Meredith, J. Transurethral operations employing high-frequency currents in patients with demand cardiac pacemakers. *J.Urol.* 1972, 108: 446–448.

Hauser, R.C. Status report: interference in modern pacemakers. *Medtronic News* 1994, 22(1): 12–20.

Hayes, D.L., Wang, P.J., Reynolds, D.W., et al. Interference with cardiac pacemakers with cellular telephones. *N. Engl. J. Med.* 1997, 336(21): 1473–1479.

International Electrotechnical Commission, Geneva, Switzerland. Documents available from Global Engineering Documents, Clayton, MO 63105.

Jenkins, J.M. and Woody, J.A. Cardiac pacemaker responses to power frequency signals. IEEE Int. Symp. on Electromagnetic Compatibility. *IEEE* 1978: 273–277.

Jenkins, J.M. and Caswell, S.A. Detection algorithms in implantable cardioverter defibrillation. *Proc. IEEE* 1996, 84(3): 428–445.

Karson, T.H., Grace, K., and Denes, F. Stereo speaker silences automatic implanted cardioverter defibrillator. *N. Engl. J. Med.* 1989, 320(24): 1628–1629.

Kaye, G.C., Butros, G.S., Allen, A., et al. The effect of external electrical interference on implanted cardiac pacemakers. *PACE* 1988, 11: 999–1008.

Khastgir, T., Aarons, D., and Veltri, E. Sudden bradyarrhythmic death in patients with the implanted cardioverter defibrillator: report of two cases. *PACE* 1991, 14: 395–398.

Kim, S.G., Furman, S.G., Matos, J.A., et al. Automatic implantable cardioverter defibrillator inadvertent discharges during permanent pacemaker magnet tests. *PACE* 1987, 10(Part 1): 579–582.

Kim, S.G., Furman, S., Waspe, L., et al. Pacer artifacts induced failure of an automatic implanted cardioverter defibrillator to detect ventricular fibrillation. *Am. J. Cardiol.* 1986, 57: 880–881.

Knutson, T. and Bulkeley, W.M. Stray Signals. *Wall Street Journal* June 15,1994.

Lau, F.Y.K., Billiteh, M., and Wintroub, H.J. Protection of implanted pacemakers from excessive electrical energy of defibrillation shock. *Am. J. Cardiol.* 1969, 23: 244–249.

Leahy, W.R., Messimino, R.J., and Wohlfert, W.J. Intermittent failure of a Stockert/Shiley multiflow roller pump. *J. Extracoporeal Technol.* 1993, 25(1): 74–77.

Lerner, S.M. Suppression of a demand pacemaker by transurethral electrocautery. *Anesth. Analg. Current Res.* 1973, 52(5): 703–706.

Levine, P.A., Barrold, S.S., Fletcher, R.D., et al. Adverse acute and chronic effects of electrical defibrillation and cardioversion on implanted unipolar cardiac pacing systems. *J. Am. Coll. Cardiol.* 1983, 1(6): 1413–1422.

Lichter, L. and Borrie, J. Radio-frequency hazards with cardiac pacemakers. *Br. Med. J.* 1965,1: 1513–1518.

Marco, D., Eisinger, G., and Hayes, D.L. Testing a work environment for electromagnetic interference. *PACE* 1992, 15: 2016–2022.

Martin, R. Designing for compliance: immunity to ESD. *Compliance Eng.* 1993, 10: 13–21.

McCarty, R.J. and Glasser, S.P. The arrhythmogenic effect of static electricity on the dog heart. *Am. Heart J.* 1977, 93(4): 496–500.

Mirowski, M. et al. The development of the transvenous automatic defibrillator. *Arch. Intern. Med.* 1972, 129: 773–779.

Mirowski, M. et al. Feasibility and effectiveness of low-energy catheter defibrillation in man. *Circulation* 1972, 47: 79–85.

Naegeli, B. and Burkart, F. Intermittent pacemaker malfunction caused by digital mobile telephones. *J. Am. Coll. Cardiol.* 1996, 27: 1471–1477.

National Fire Protection Association, 470 Atlantic Avenue, Boston, MA 07210. National Electrical Code (NFPA #70), Essential Electrical Systems for Hospitals (NFPA #76).

Nowak, B., Roscona, S., Noff, C., et al. Is there risk for interaction between mobile phones and single-lead VDD pacemakers? Abstracts 45th Ann. Sci. Session ACC. *J. Am. Coll. Cardiol.* 1996, 27(2): 236A.

O'Donoghue, J. K. Inhibition of a demand pacemaker by electrosurgery. *Chest* 1973, 64(5): 664–665.

Pride, H.B. and McKinley, D.E. Third-degree burns from the use of an external cardiac pacing device. *Crit. Care Med.* 1990, 18: 572–573.

Ruggera, P. and O'Bryan, E.R. Studies of apnea monitor radiofrequency electromagnetic interference. *Int Conf. IEEE EMBS* 1991, 13(4): 1641–1643.

Ruggera, P.S., O'Bryan, R., and Casamiento, J.P. Automated radiofrequency electromagnetic interference testing on apnea monitors using an open area test site. *Proc. IEEE EMBS Conf.* 1992, 2839–2840.

Rustan, P.L., Hunt, W.D., and Mitchell, J.C. Microwave oven interference with cardiac pacemakers. *Med. Instr.* 1973, 7: 185–188.

Schmitt, C., Brachmann, J., Waldecker, B., et al. Implantable cardioverter defibrillator: possible hazards of electromagnetic interference. *PACE* 1991, 14: 982–984.

Silberberg, J.L. Performance degradation of electronic medical devices due to electromagnetic interference. *Compliance Eng.* 1993, Fall: 1–8.

Silbert, P.L., Roth, P.A., Kanz, B.S., et al. Interference from cellular telephones in the electroencephalogram. *J. Polysomnog. Technol.* 1994, December: 20–22.

Smith, R.B. and Wise, W.S. Pacemaker malfunction from urethral electrocautery. *J.A.M.A.* 1971, 218: 256.

Spotnitz, H.M., Ott, G.Y., Begger, J.T., et al. Methods of implantable cardioverter-defibrillator pacemaker insertion to avoid interactions. *Ann. Thor. Surg.* 1992, 53: 253–257.

Titel, J.H. and El Etr, A.A. Fibrillation resulting from pacemaker electrodes and electrocautery during surgery. *Anesthesiology* 1968, 29(4): 845–846.

Valentinuzzi, M.E., Geddes, L.A., and Baker, L.E. The law of impedance pneumography. *Med. Biol. Eng.* 1971, 9: 157–163.

Wajsczuk, W., Mowry, F.M., and Dugan, N.L. Deactivation of a demand pacemaker by transurethral electrosurgery. *N. Engl. J. Med.* 1969, 280(1): 34–35.

Witters, D. Medical device EMI: the CDRH perspective. AAMI Conf. on Electromagnetic Compatibility for Medical Devices 1995, *AAMI Conf. Rep.* pp. 7–23.

Zoll, P.M., Zoll, R.H., and Belgard, A.H. External noninvasive electrical stimulation of the heart. *Crit. Care Med.* 1981, 9(5): 393–394.

Zoll, P.M. Resuscitation of the heart in ventricular standstill by external electric stimulation. *N. Engl. J. Med.* 1952, 247: 768–771.

3 Electrosurgery

CONTENTS

INTRODUCTION

Electrosurgery employs 0.5 to 2 MHz (alternating) radiofrequency current applied to a small-area (active) electrode to produce desiccation, coagulation, and cutting in living tissue. Although Cushing and Bovie (1928) are usually credited with popularizing electrosurgery, it was in use much earlier. In 1911, Clark, in the U.S., developed a spark-gap generator and used its alternating current to remove skin blemishes. However, Doyen (1909), in France, had used a similar unit to excise skin blemishes. By 1930, the advantages of electrosurgical techniques were recognized; among these are the saving of time, assurance of asepsis, absence of bleeding, and elimination of the transfer of infection from diseased to normal tissue that sometimes occurred with a scalpel. Wound healing with electrodissection is almost the same as with scalpel cuts. These features were testified to by a panel of eminent surgeons who were convened on the occasion of the Conference on Electrosurgery at the Clinical Congress of the American College of Surgeons (1931). The enthusiasm in these reports, which cover a wide range of surgical procedures, shows how quickly surgeons embraced the new techniques. At this conference there was a report on wound healing (Ellis, 1931), in which it was shown that, except for skin incisions, there is little difference between scalpel and electrosurgical cutting methods. Shortly thereafter, the first American textbook on electrosurgery was published by Kelly and Ward (1932); in it there is a good review of the histologic changes in tissue in response to electrosurgical currents. Earlier Doyen (1917) outlined his experience with the spark-gap electrosurgical unit.

The electrosurgical instrument is a generator of controlled radiofrequency (rf) current that is applied to an active point, blade, ball, or loop electrode to produce the desired thermal tissue response.

The terminology associated with electrosurgery is not always precise. Terms such as cautery, electrocautery, surgical diathermy, and Bovie are in common use. The following definitions of these terms will serve as a guide to use of the correct term. A cautery is a heated rod (like a poker) used to cut and coagulate tissue; its origin is in Arabic medicine. An electrocautery is an electrically heated rod, not unlike a soldering iron, which can indeed be used to cut and coagulate tissue. Surgical diathermy is an older term that is used in the U.K. to designate the use of high-frequency current in surgery. The term "Bovie" is used almost interchangeably with an electrosurgical unit because it was W.T. Bovie who built the first practical (spark-gap) electrosurgical unit that was introduced to medicine in 1928 by Cushing and Bovie (see Geddes et al., 1977, for the history of electrosurgery). Because modern electrosurgical units no longer contain spark gaps or vacuum tubes to generate the cutting and coagulating currents, the correct term for the generator of high-frequency current for surgery is an electrosurgical unit (ESU).

Figure 1 is a sketch of the three components of an electrosurgical system: (1) the hand-held probe (active electrode), (2) the electrosurgical unit (ESU), and (3) the dispersive electrode. It is at the probe tip, which may or may not be in contact with the tissue, where the three processes (desiccation, coagulation, and cutting) occur.

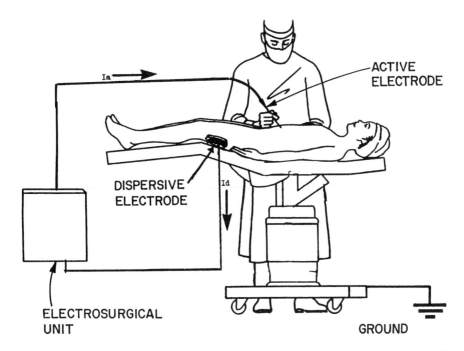

FIGURE 1   The three components of an electrosurgical system: (1) the active electrode, (2) the dispersive electrode, and (3) the electrosurgical unit (ESU).

Figure 1 depicts the use of a monopolar active electrode which has a small area; consequently, the current density is high and heating occurs thereunder. Note that the dispersive electrode is very large so that the current is dispersed widely to avoid skin heating. In normal operation the current (I_a) leaving the ESU passes through the active electrode and enters the body. The return current (I_d) from the dispersive electrode is equal to I_a and returns to the ESU. The subject of alternate current paths and the bipolar electrode will be discussed subsequently. The ESU is under the control of the surgeon either by buttons on the active electrode or by a double footswitch.

It is important to note that the large-area dispersive electrode provides a safe return path for the electrosurgical current. It is useful to recognize that heating depends on current density (mA/cm²) squared and the duration of current flow. Therefore, the maximum heating occurs under the tip of the small-area, hand-held probe electrode. The dispersive electrode is designed so that negligible skin heating occurs thereunder. There is a performance standard for dispersive electrodes.

ELECTRODES

Both monopolar and bipolar electrodes are used. The monopolar electrode will be discussed first. A variety of electrode tips are used to deliver desiccating, coagulating, and cutting current. These tips are plugged into the pencil-like holder held by the

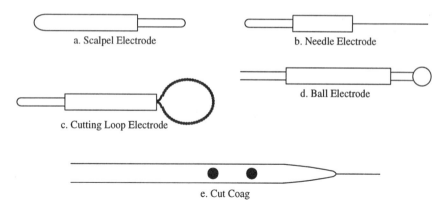

FIGURE 2 Monopolar electrodes.

surgeon. Figure 2A illustrates the standard blade (scalpel) tip which is flat, smooth, and not sharp like a scalpel blade. Smooth cutting is produced by vaporization of the cells in contact with the tip as it is advanced through tissue. The speed of cutting is determined by the intensity of the cutting current. The needle electrode, shown in Figure 2B, is inserted into the tissue and is used for desiccation and coagulation. The cutting loop (Figure 2C) is used to excise warts, polyps, and tumors. The ball electrode (Figure 2D) is used to provide a broad area of fulguration, (i.e., sparking), as is often used in treating skin blemishes (fulgur = lightning).

In Figure 2E is shown an active electrode with two push buttons; one allows delivery of cutting current and the other permits delivery of coagulating current. Such hand-held probes come packaged and sterilized and are disposable items. With most ESU units, a dual foot switch allows delivery of these currents to the hand-held active electrode.

Figure 3 illustrates a bipolar electrode. No dispersive electrode is required because the tissue to be coagulated is grasped between the tips of two active electrodes. The arms of the older bipolar electrodes were uninsulated; modern bipolar electrodes carry insulation down to near the tip. Activation of the bipolar electrode is via depressing the foot pedal controller. Note that the current is confined to the region between the electrode tips.

DISPERSIVE ELECTRODES

The dispersive (sometimes called the Bovie pad, patient plate, ground, or indifferent) electrode provides a safe return path for the electrosurgical current. The electrode area is large enough so that there is negligible heating of the skin thereunder. Typically, the dispersive electrode is placed over a fleshy part of the body; it is never placed over a bony prominence because there is the risk of uneven current distribution which could produce a hot spot or a burn.

There are two types of dispersive electrode: (1) conductive and (2) capacitive. The conductive type establishes ohmic (resistive) contact with the subject; the capacitive type does not. The capacitive electrode consists of a metal plate covered

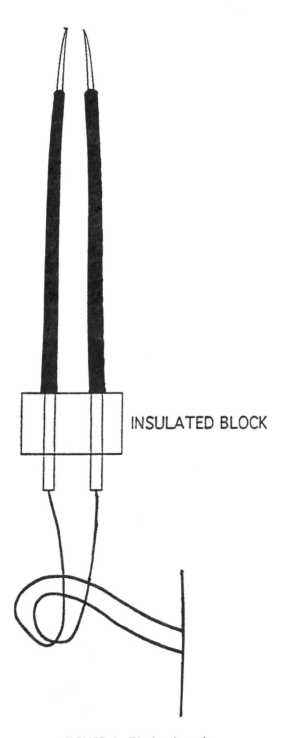

FIGURE 3 Bipolar electrode.

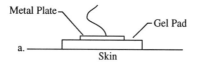

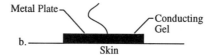

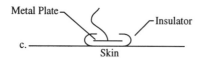

FIGURE 4 Dispersive electrodes.

by insulating film (dielectric). In this way one "plate" of the capacitor is the subject, the other is the metal within the electrode.

CONDUCTIVE DISPERSIVE ELECTRODES

The first dispersive electrodes consisted of a large-area, bare, dry metal plate on which the patient lay. Variable contact area led to the use of flexible metal foil, insulated on the back and surrounded by an adhesive perimeter which allowed placement of the electrode at any convenient body site. The temperature distribution under a dry metal-plate electrode on human skin was reported by Pearce et al. (1978) and Geddes et al. (1980). Such dry electrodes are rarely used nowadays.

To improve contact with the skin, an electrolytic gel is used with metal-foil dispersive electrodes. A peel-off cover protects the electrode during storage. The skin-temperature distribution of a typical gelled metal-foil electrode was reported by Pearce et al. (1978) and Geddes et al. (1979).

In some dispersive electrodes, the electrolytic gel is incorporated into a foam pad that bridges the gap between the metal foil and skin; Figure 4A illustrates the essential components. A peel-off cover protects the electrode in storage. The temperature distribution is similar to that for the gelled metal-foil electrode.

Advances in adhesive technology resulted in the ability to include an electrolyte and thereby create a conducting adhesive dispersive electrode. Such an electrode is shown in Figure 4B and consists of a metal foil, backed by an insulator with an adhesive perimeter. The conducting adhesive sticks to the metal foil and a peel-off cover exposes the conducting adhesive which embraces the skin well.

Irrespective of design, the conductive dispersive electrode makes ohmic (resistive) contact with the subject. The current distribution under such an electrode is not uniform, the current density under the perimeter being several times higher than under the center of the electrode (Caruso et al., 1979; Overmeyer et al., 1979).

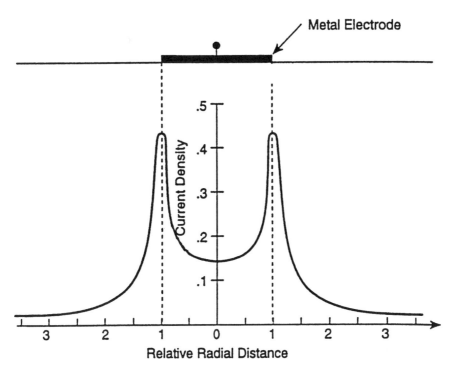

FIGURE 5 Current density on the skin under a conducting dispersive electrode. (Redrawn from Caruso, P., Pearce, J.A., and DeWitt, D.P. *Proc. 7th N. Engl. Bioeng. Conf.* 1979, 373–374; and Overmeyer, K., Pearce, J.A., and DeWitt, D.P. *Trans. ASME* 1979, 191: 66–72.

Because heating depends on current-density squared, the skin under the perimeter of a conducting electrode is warmer than the skin under the center of the electrode; Figure 5 illustrates this point.

CAPACITIVE DISPERSIVE ELECTRODE

Because the frequency (f) of electrosurgical current is high, it is possible to cover the metal foil with a thin insulating (dielectric) film; Figure 4C illustrates the principle. The capacitance (C) depends on the electrode area (A), dielectric constant (k), and inversely with the thickness (t) of the dielectric film. C = kA/t. The size (area) of the electrode is chosen so that the reactance (½πfC) of the capacitance is sufficiently small that an adequate return path is established with the subject. As with the other dispersive electrodes, an insulating back and adhesive perimeter are provided and a peel-off cover protects the dielectric surface during storage.

Two features distinguish the capacitive electrode from all other types: (1) there is no ohmic (resistive) contact with the subject, and (2) the skin-temperature distribution is more uniform than that for conductive dispersive electrodes, this being the nature of a capacitive interface (Pearce, 1986). The skin-temperature distribution for capacitive dispersive electrodes was reported by Pearce et al. (1980).

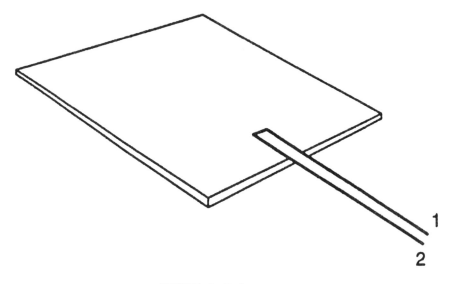

FIGURE 6   Patient sentry.

DISPERSIVE ELECTRODE MONITORS

Because of the hazard of alternate-current path burns if a dispersive electrode is not connected to the ESU or becomes partially or totally dislodged, three types of dispersive electrode monitors have been developed: (1) patient sentry, (2) current comparator, and (3) patient-return monitor.

Patient Sentry

With the patient sentry the dispersive electrode (Figure 6) is connected to the ESU by two conductors (1, 2). A circuit within the ESU prevents delivery of current unless there is continuity between conductors 1 and 2. In the earlier ESUs, a relay was held closed by the continuity measured between conductors 1 and 2. The patient sentry was first incorporated into the Bovie CSV units. Newer ESUs use an SCR (silicon-controlled rectifier) to allow delivery of electrosurgical current only when continuity is verified; an alarm is sounded if not.

Although a useful safety method, such dispersive electrodes with two conductors can only be connected to an ESU with the patient sentry feature. Such a patient sentry provides no information on whether or not the dispersive electrode is applied to the subject; it only informs that the electrode is connected to the ESU.

Current Comparator

Referring to Figure 1, it is obvious that the magnitude of the current (Ia) flowing through the active electrode is the same as the current (Id) flowing through the dispersive electrode. If the dispersive electrode becomes dislodged and an alternate current path to ground is established by the patient, Ia will be larger than Id.

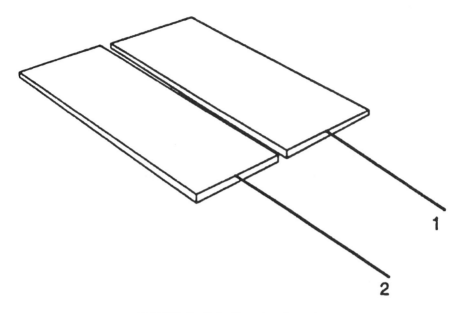

FIGURE 7 Split dispersive electrode.

Therefore, by comparing the magnitudes of Ia and Id, it is possible to identify the existence of an alternate current path and automatically disable the output of an ESU and sound an alarm. This type of current comparator is embodied in some ESUs.

Patient-Return Monitor

A different type of electrode monitor was developed by Valleylab, Inc. and uses a split dispersive electrode, as shown schematically in Figure 7. When the electrode is applied to the patient, a circuit in the ESU monitors the impedance between conductors 1 and 2. When the split electrode is on the patient, the impedance between electrodes 1 and 2 is low. If the ESU senses a high impedance between conductors 1 and 2, it means that the dispersive electrode has not been applied properly, or has not been applied to the patient; therefore, the ESU is inhibited from delivering current and an alarm is sounded. Note that this type of monitor identifies (1) connection of the electrode to the ESU, (2) proper application of the electrode to the patient, and (3) continuity of the two conductors leading to the ESU. To obtain the advantages of the split dispersive electrode requires the use of an ESU designed for use of such an electrode.

PERFORMANCE STANDARDS

As stated previously, the function of a dispersive electrode is to provide a safe return path for the electrosurgical current. The area of the electrode must be large enough so that excessive skin heating does not occur. There is a performance standard (AAMI HF 18-R-2/93) being developed. Briefly, it states that the skin-temperature rise must not exceed 6°C for a 700-mA (rms) current applied for 60 sec. The standard should be consulted for the methods for testing.

TYPES OF CURRENT

Two types of radio-frequency current (unmodulated and modulated) are used to induce the three types of tissue response (desiccation, coagulation, and cutting). Moreover, there are two techniques for applying the hand-held probe, also called the active electrode or pencil: one brings the tip of the probe in contact with the tissue, then the ESU is activated. The other technique brings the tip of the probe in close proximity to the tissue; then the ESU is activated and an arc carries the current to the tissue. Which technique is used depends on the desired tissue response.

Figure 8 illustrates the current waveforms for cutting and coagulation. In general, cutting is achieved with continuous, i.e., unmodulated current; Figures 8A and 8B illustrate the type of current used for cutting. The waveform in Figure 8A is produced by the older push–pull type of vacuum-tube units. The radio frequency cutting current is delivered in 1/120-half-sinusoidal bursts. In the newer solid-state units the current is more constant, as shown in Figure 8B.

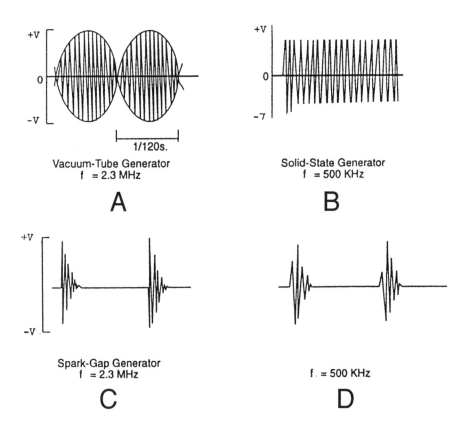

FIGURE 8 Electrosurgical current waveforms.

TABLE 1
Current Used in Electrosurgical Procedures

Procudure	Current[a] (mA) Min	Max	Avg	Duration of activation (sec) Min	Max	Avg
Transurethral resection						
Cut	239 (162)	407 (297)	297 (200)	1.6 (0.68)	3.8 (2.3)	2.1 (0.69)
Coag	179 (78)	419 (400)	256 (88)	1.4 (0.5)	5 (7.6)	1.9 (0.7)
Laparoscopic tubal ligation						
Cut	126 (120)	430 (290)	239 (135)	1.7 (0.58)	5.4 (4.9)	2.6 (3.2)
Coag	61 (57)	118 (80)	86 (70)	3.2 (0.31)	26 (20)	10 (7.4)
General surgery[b]						
Cut	238 (188)	340 (101)	281 (147)	2 (2)	7.6 (11)	2.2 (1.8)
Coag	146 (94)	267 (157)	198 (114)	4.7 (5.2	11 (7.8)	6.5 (5.2)

[a] Numbers in parentheses are standard deviations.

[b] General surgical procedures include prostatectimy, laparotomy, thoracotomy, hip pinning, hysterectomy, nephrectomy, and D&C.

Courtesy of J. DeRosa, NDM Co., Dayton, OH.

The coagulating current waveforms are shown in Figures 8C and 8D. Note that in both cases the duty cycle is short. Figure 8C illustrates the coagulating waveform provided by the older spark-gap (Bovie) generators and the bursts of radio-frequency current are delivered at 120/sec. Figure 8D illustrates the coagulating waveform provided by the newer solid-state units which deliver the bursts at typically 20,000/sec. Table 1 presents the current levels and activation times used for different surgical procedures.

Electrosurgical current is low in frequency when one considers the "skin effect", which describes the manner in which high-frequency current crowds to the periphery of a conductor. Skin effect for tissues is discussed in the chapter on electromagnetic interference (EMI).

ISOLATED-OUTPUT ELECTROSURGICAL UNIT

An isolated output circuit is defined as one with no ohmic contact and low leakage capacitance to ground. This is achieved with a transformer, the secondary winding providing the isolated voltage source; Figure 9A illustrates this scheme and Figure 9B shows the equivalent circuit in which the distributed capacitance (C) has been gathered and represented as C1 and C2. Note that although there is no ohmic connection to ground on the isolated output, there is distributed capacitance (C1, C2) to ground and therefore the degree of isolation from ground depends on the magnitude of these capacitances.

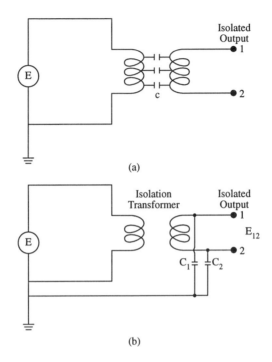

FIGURE 9 Isolated output circuit.

Many modern electrosurgical units have an isolating transformer that delivers the electrosurgical current to the active and dispersive electrodes. Contact with any grounded object and one side of the isolated output should cause little current to flow. However, electrosurgical current has a frequency ranging from 0.5 to 2 MHz; therefore, the effect of the distributed capacitance is not negligible and some current will flow in a conductor connected between one side of the isolated output and ground; the conductor could be a subject.

To demonstrate that current can flow through a conductor connected to one side of the output of an isolated ESU and ground, Finlay et al. (1974) measured the current for different values of resistance (R) connected between ground and one side of the output of an isolated-output ESU. The current was measured for different ESU output settings using cutting current; Figure 10 presents his results. Note that a substantial current can flow to ground.

Many manufacturers specify the quality of isolation in teams of a power ratio (P2/P1), where P1 is the output power delivered to a 1000-ohm noninductive resistor connected across the output terminals of the isolated ESU and P2 is the leakage power delivered to a 1000-ohm resistor connected between ground and one side of the isolated output of the ESU; Figure 11 illustrates the test circuit and measurements are usually made with the ESU delivering cutting current at half-maximum output setting. According to Finlay et al. (1974), a typical value for P2/P1 is about 0.5%. Note that this test describes the performance of the ESU without patient cables attached.

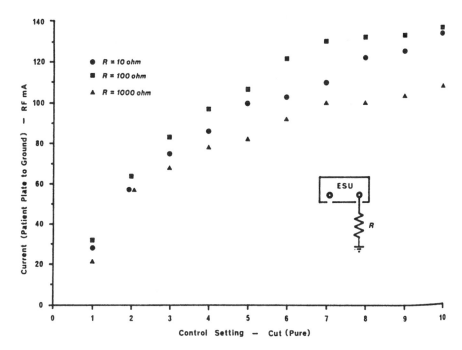

FIGURE 10 Current to ground through R vs. output setting for an isolated output ESU. (Redrawn from Finlay, B., Couchie, D., Boyce, L., et al. *Anesthesiology* 1974, 41(3): 263–269.)

The importance of this leakage current with an isolated-output ESU was demonstrated by Finlay et al. (1974), who described a burn under an ECG electrode on a small child undergoing electrosurgery for a neurosurgical procedure. The effective electrode skin-contact area was 5 mm², resulting in a current density of 9.1 mA/mm², a current density above burn threshold, as Finlay et al. demonstrated by a dog study.

Although reducing the hazards of electrosurgery, the isolated-output ESU can be associated with accidents. There are two situations that can arise which could result in a patient burn. The first pertains to activation of the ESU with the active monopolar electrode not contacting the subject (i.e., the electrode is in a holster) and with a dispersive electrode on the patient and connected to the ESU. In this case, the patient is exposed to the high open-circuit voltage of the ESU and the return path can be via any grounded object that contacts the patient. The leakage capacitance to ground in the ESU completes the circuit.

The second situation in which an isolated output ESU can produce a patient burn occurs when the dispersive electrode is on the patient but not plugged into the ESU and the activated monopolar active electrode contacts the patient. Therefore, the high open-circuit ESU voltage is applied to the patient. The return path is via any grounded object in contact with the patient. The remainder of the return path to ground is via the capacitance to ground in the ESU.

In the two foregoing situations the current will not be large if the capacitance to ground in the isolated ISU is small. However, this potential hazard should be recognized.

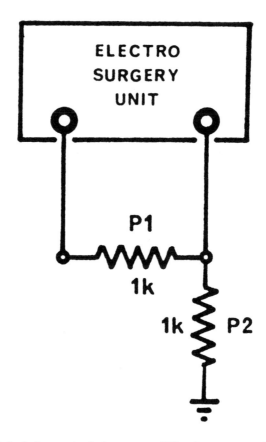

FIGURE 11   Method of measuring leakage power (P2) and output power (P1) for an isolated-output ESU. (Redrawn from Finlay, B., Couchie, D., Boyce, L., et al. *Anesthesiology* 1974, 41(3): 263–269.)

A less common, but dangerous, situation can arise if the active monopolar electrode is in contact with ground and the ESU is activated when a dispersive electrode is on the subject and connected to the ESU. In this situation, the patient is raised to the open-circuit voltage of the ESU and arcing can occur from the patient to a nearly grounded object, thereby causing a burn.

Whether any of the foregoing potential accidents will occur depends on the type of alarm that is associated with an ESU and the dispersive electrode. Such accidents are unlikely with newer ESUs, but a large number of older units are still in use.

TISSUE RESPONSES

CUTTING

Surgical cutting (Figure 12A) employs unmodulated radio-frequency current of the type shown in Figures 8A and 8B. The tip of the probe is brought into contact with the tissue surface and the ESU is activated. An arc is struck and the tissue vaporizes,

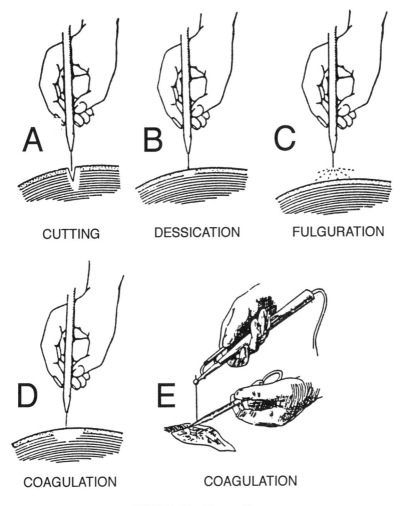

CUTTING   DESSICATION   FULGURATION

COAGULATION   COAGULATION

FIGURE 12 Tissue effects.

producing a scalpel-like cut; the permissible speed of cutting depends on the current intensity. However, the lips of the incision usually bleed and coagulation current is used to arrest the bleeding. In many ESUs, it is possible to combine (blend) cutting and coagulating current electrically so that coagulation accompanies cutting.

Honig (1975) has shown that the temperature at the tip of the electrode is high enough to boil tissue fluid, which causes the cells to burst. The arc represents a very localized source of heat so that the cutting is highly localized. In addition, the arc represents ionized gas (plasma), which has a low resistance. Therefore, as the cutting electrode is advanced, it is surrounded by steam and hot ionized gas which emits light.

DESICCATION

Desiccation (Figure 12B), i.e., drying, is produced by placing the tip of the probe in contact with the tissue and activating the ESU. Low current (of either type) can be used; no arc is formed and the fluid is driven from the tissue surrounding the probe tip.

COAGULATION

Coagulation employs modulated current (Figure 8C and 8D) and several different techniques are employed with the active electrode. With spray coagulation (Figure 12C), sometimes called fulguration (fulgur = lightning), the active electrode is brought close to the tissue and the ESU is activated. Arcs travel from the tip of the probe to the tissue, each arc striking a different site, the result being a more-or-less circular area of coagulation. This technique is used to remove skin blemishes and sometimes to close very small bleeding vessels. Alternately, the active electrode is placed in contact with the bleeder (Figure 12D) and the ESU is activated; no arcing occurs and the tissue temperature rises to above 45°C. White coagulation is the term used when lower current and longer times are used. The tissue is dehydrated slowly and becomes whitish.

Another technique for closing larger blood vessels was developed by Ward (1925) and is shown in Figure 12E. The bleeder is grasped with a hemostat or forceps to arrest bleeding; then the tip of the active electrode is touched to the hemostat and the ESU is activated. No arc is formed and either type of current can be used to seal the bleeder. The surgeon's gloves provide insulation for the hands.

The ESU must never be activated while holding a hemostat (or metal instrument) which is in contact with the active electrode while the instrument is not in contact with the tissue, because the open-circuit voltage of an ESU is high and could break down the insulation of the glove and burn or shock the surgeon. The breakdown voltage for rubber is 300 V/1000th in. (mil). The breakdown for a typical plastic is 300 to 1000 V/mil of thickness.

ARGON-ENHANCED COAGULATION

McGreevy and Bertrand (1988) found that the forcible passage of argon gas through a hollow electrode during coagulation not only cleared the field, but the gas became ionized and produced a flexible eschar with uniform depth and absence of charring. The ionized gas at the electrode tip is very uniform in extent, easy to manipulate, and coagulates very well on highly vascularized tissue, such as the liver. Other than the special hollow electrode and means for controlling the flow of argon, standard electrosurgical fulgurating current is used. The hazards associated with this technology are no different than those with conventional open electrosurgery.

CURRENT CROWDING

Even with everything operating properly, there are situations in which there is a risk of injury resulting from electrosurgical current crowding, i.e., a condition in which the return-path current is forced to flow through tissue with a small cross-sectional area. Mitchell and Lumb (1966) use the term "channeling" for this situation. Perhaps the best way to illustrate current crowding is to consider first a no current-crowding

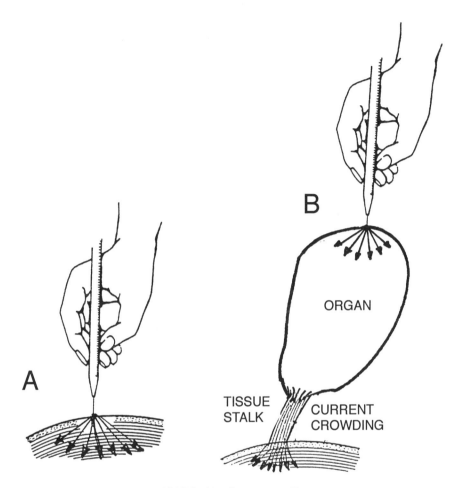

FIGURE 13 Current crowding.

example. Figure 13A illustrates an active electrode delivering electrosurgical current to a tissue. Note that the current spreads radially from the small-area entry site (active electrode); therefore, all of the heating is at this site. The bulk of the tissue and blood flow constitute a heat sink.

Figure 13B illustrates the application of electrosurgical current to an organ connected to the body by a slender stalk, which might be a duct, nerve, artery, and/or vein. Observe that the electrosurgical current spreads radially from the active electrode tip. All of this current is forced to reach the dispersive electrode via the tissue stalk, which has a small cross-sectional area and therefore a high electrical resistance. Because the heating is proportional to the current density (amps/cm^2) squared, the resistance and the duration of current flow, the opportunity for coagulating the stalk is high. Mitchell and Lumb (1966) and Schellhammer (1974) recognized this hazard. Mitchell and Lumb stated:

The example of this condition (channeling) most commonly occurring is in operations on the testis and scrotum (e.g., hydrocele), when the spermatic cord and its vessels channel the whole of the operating current. In these circumstances the narrow pedicle formed by the cord may concentrate sufficient heat to thrombose all the blood-vessels, resulting in necrosis of the organ.

Current-crowding accidents are described elsewhere in this chapter.

COMPLICATIONS WITH ELECTROSURGICAL CURRENT

Electrosurgical current can be a source of electromagnetic interference (EMI) and cause environmental and implanted devices to malfunction; these cases are discussed in the chapter on EMI. Muscle stimulation is by no means rare with electrosurgery; these cases are discussed in this chapter. Accidental burns are all too common; these will be discussed in this chapter. Finally, the inappropriate use of electrosurgery in the presence of a flammable material and oxygen constitutes a fire hazard; these accidents are discussed in the chapter on anesthesia and in this chapter.

MUSCLE CONTRACTION

Skeletal-muscle contraction is not uncommon during electrosurgery and can present a hazard in some circumstances. For example, Prentiss et al. (1965), referring to transurethral resection, stated:

> It is estimated that the adductor contraction occurs in 1 of 5 patients with large intraurethral prostatic adenomas or laterally placed vesical neoplasms.
>
> The obturator nerve stimulation occurs when the prostatic capsule or deeper muscular layers of the bladder are approached. The adductor muscle contraction develops so suddenly that perforation may be unavoidable and leads to extravasation. It always deters the completion of the operation and dissemination of tumor cells is a distinct possibility.

To avoid adductor muscle contraction during transurethral resection, Prentiss et al. (1965) recommended the use of nerve block or myoneural-junction block. Interestingly, they noted that the cutting current provided by their ESU was modulated at 120/sec (Figure 8A). They developed an unmodulated ESU operating at 3.601 MHz, but still encountered muscle contraction and concluded that the presence of a cutting arc generated low-frequency currents that produced the stimulation, a fact that was proved much later.

MECHANISM OF MUSCLE STIMULATION

Foster and Geddes (1986) devised a simple experiment designed to test the ability of electrosurgical current to stimulate the dog sciatic nerve with and without an arc at the tip of the electrosurgical probe, which was remote from the nerve, as shown in Figure 14. The active electrosurgical electrode was placed over a saline-soaked sponge in a metal dish which was connected to a gauze-covered, saline-soaked

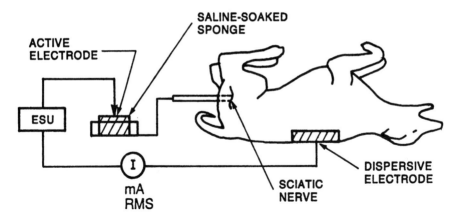

FIGURE 14 Method of demonstrating muscle stimulation with electrosurgical current. (Redrawn from Foster, K.S. and Geddes, L.A. *Med. Instrum.* 1986, 20(6): 335–336.)

electrode applied to the exposed sciatic nerve of an anesthetized dog. A conventional dispersive electrosurgical electrode provided the return path to the ESU. Thus, the electrosurgical current could be applied with or without an arc by selecting the position of the tip of the active electrode (e.g., above the sponge or advanced into it), as shown in Figure 14.

Stimulation of the sciatic nerve causes contraction of the gastrocnemius muscle and rotates the foot (downward) around the ankle joint. Therefore, if any pulsating current flowed in the circuit, the sciatic nerve would be stimulated, thereby contracting the gastrocnemius muscle.

Two types of experiment were performed. One consisted of applying electrosurgical current with no arc, i.e., the tip of the active electrode was plunged into the sponge before the ESU was activated; the other employed activation of the ESU with the tip of the active electrode just above the sponge and slowly advancing it until an arc was struck. Thus, the current that flowed represented the no-arc and arc conditions. The rms current (I) was measured in both cases with a thermocouple-type ammeter. Table 2 summarizes the results and shows that with no arc, in only one case was there a trace of muscle contraction. In all cases with an arc, muscle contraction occurred.

It has been shown by Pearce et al. (1986) and Tucker et al. (1984) that the presence of an arc in the path of electrosurgical current produces low-frequency components capable of stimulation. That the cause of muscle contraction during electrosurgery is due mainly to stimulation of motor nerves comes from two sources: (1) the muscle contraction can be distant from the site of the active electrosurgical electrode and (2) nerve blockade and myoneural blocking agents block muscle contraction.

In addition to adductor muscle contraction during transurethral resection, other muscles have been observed to contract during electrosurgery; the following is an example.

Geddes and Moore (1990) reported the following accident that resulted from muscle contractions during electrosurgery:

TABLE 2
The Stimulating Capabilities of Cutting
and Coagulating Current

Instrument No.	Mode	Current [mA (rms)]	Contraction Arc	Contraction No Arc
1	Coag.	200	Yes	No
	Cut	500	Yes	No
2	Pure cut	200	Yes	No
	Spark gap coag.	600	—	No
	(mod. hemo.)	200	Yes	—
	Spark gap coag.	500	—	No
	(marked hemo.)	100	Yes	—
	Spark gap coag.	250	—	Trace
	(max. hemo.)	<100	Yes	

A 32-year-old white male with tender enlarged lymph nodes in the left posterior cervical triangle presented to the office of a general surgeon. There was also a 25 to 30-pound weight loss over a two to three-month period. He was hospitalized for diagnostic studies which were negative. Suspecting possible Hodgkin's disease, he was taken to the operating room for removal of the largest node. When the surgeon encountered a small bleeder in the subcutaneous fat, he used a standard, solid-state electrosurgical unit in the monopolar mode with a coagulation at a setting between 3 or 4 to stop the bleeding. As the bleeder was approached with the active electrode to perform coagulation, the patient experienced a severe jolt which he likened to being shocked by an electric outlet. The operative report made no reference to the incident or the electrosurgical unit, stating only that "A nerve, presumably of the cervical plexus was anesthetized and retracted posteriorly and the subjacent node was dissected out." The discharge summary, however, noted that "during this operation, while in the subcutaneous tissue under local anesthesia, a standard ESU was used to coagulate a small bleeding blood vessel and this caused a rather violent jerk in the patient's left leg and left arm. The ESU was used no further during the operation. As the operation continued, the accessory nerve was noted to be near the area and it was presumed that the stimulation of a nerve is what caused this violent spasm.

The surgeon was concerned that the ESU had malfunctioned. Although the machine used in the procedure was not identified, all machines were checked approximately 2 months after the operation and all were reported to be functioning normally. The disposable active electrode and grounding pad were not retained.

Subsequent to the operation, the patient complained of pain in the neck, left arm, and shoulder. When seen in the physician's office 3 days later, he was unable to completely abduct his left arm. An electromyographic study 18 days after surgery revealed "moderately severe denervation of the rhomboids, levator scapulae, supra-spinatus, infra-spinatus, and trapezius muscles," prompting the neurologist to note that the results "may provide evidence of involvement of the nerve to the trapezius, dorsal scapular nerve, and supra-scapular nerve. This may be secondary to partial injury to the upper brachial plexus on the left."

> Approximately one month after surgery, the surgeon was concerned that the patient exhibited diffuse atrophy of his deltoids and other shoulder girdle muscles. Subsequent orthopedic treatment resulted in a conclusion of a dual lesion: brachial plexus injury and cervical disc degeneration at C5-6, the latter resulting in anterior intervertebral disc excisions and fusion from C4 through 7. The orthopedic surgeon felt that the patient suffered an electrical injury to the brachial plexus from direct spread of current. In addition, he doubtless had degenerative disease in his cervical spine which was not symptomatic until the violent jerking of his neck occurred. After that, the symptoms persisted until the surgery was performed on the cervical disc.

From the foregoing, it appears that the active electrosurgical electrode was near a motor nerve or plexus and that the presence of the arc produced low-frequency components that resulted in stimulation. Of the two types of electrosurgical current, the coagulating current, which is delivered in bursts, is the most likely to stimulate if an arc is struck. However, cutting (unmodulated) radio-frequency current has the potential for stimulation if an arc is struck.

EXPERIMENTAL BURN STUDIES

The most important factors in producing skin burns are contained in the burn strength-duration curve, originally presented by Moritz and Henriques (1947). This study showed that for a first-degree burn, there is a hyperbolic relationship between termperature and exposure time. Using metal chambers heated by circulating hot water, Moritz and Henriques showed that the shorter the duration of exposure, the higher the temperature required to produce irreversible epidermal injury in porcine skin, which is an excellent analog for human skin; Figure 15 presents their data. It is generally believed that a skin temperature of 45°C can cause a burn if it persists. Typically human skin temperature is about 32°C.

To identify the factors that produce an increase in skin temperature with electrosurgical current, Pearce et al. (1983) carried out controlled burn studies on pigs using 500 kHz electrosurgical current delivered to circular disk electrodes 1, 2, 4, and 8 cm applied to the backs of pigs. The skin temperature and burn severity were determined for different currents (300 to 700 mA) and times (30 to 60 sec). The skin temperature, determined thermographically, was plotted vs. the energy density factor (seconds multiplied by the square of the current density in amps/cm^2 of electrode area). Figure 16 illustrates the result; the numbers (1, 2, 3) along the abscissa identify the burn degree.

A first-degree burn is skin reddening (erythema), like a sunburn; there is no permanent skin damage. A second-degree or partial-thickness burn is characterized by blisters, vesication, and hemorrhage. A third-degree, or full-thickness burn, is characterized by zones of coagulum, denatured collagen, and brown leathery tissue called an eschar; often carbonized tissue is present. Full-thickness burns and some partial-thickness burns require skin grafting.

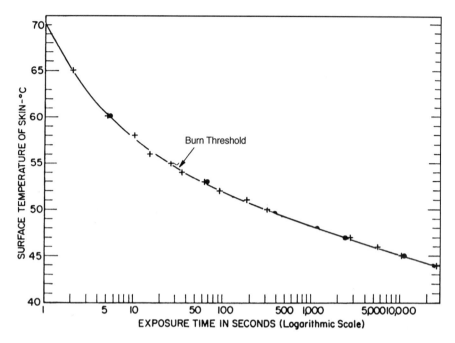

FIGURE 15   Skin temperature vs. exposure time for skin burn.   (Redrawn from Moritz, A.R. and Henriques, F.C. *Am. J. Pathol.* 1947, 23: 605–720.)

In the Pearce et al. study (1983), in general, with an energy-density factor in the range of 0.7 to 1.6 the maximum skin temperature below the electrodes was between 49 and 55°C, with single or multiple rings of second-degree burns located just inside or beyond the rim of the electrode. At all sites exposed to higher energy density (1.60 to 7.50), the maximum skin temperature beneath the electrodes was 55 to 81°C, and severe burns were produced with white to brownish, dry, firm, third-degree burns surrounded by peripheral rings of second-degree burns. No significant skin damage was produced with a skin temperature less than 45°C, representing an energy density factor of about 0.75.

DeRosa and Gadsby (1979) conducted electrosurgical burn studies with ECG electrodes and obtained data that allowed relating the skin-temperature rise to the energy density factor (seconds multiplied by current density squared). Figure 17 shows this relationship, which is in agreement with the data reported by Pearce et al. (1983) and shown in Figure 16.

ACCIDENTAL BURNS

As stated previously, the heating at an electrode site depends on the current density squared and the duration of current flow. It is useful to identify the events that occur in the absence of a satisfactory dispersive-electrode contact with the patient. In this case, the return path for the electrosurgical current will be any grounded object that the patient contacts. An example in which the dispersive electrode cable is broken

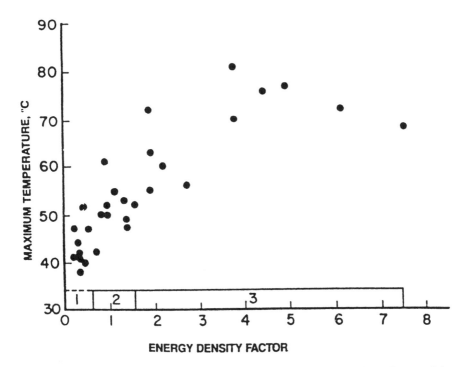

FIGURE 16 Skin-temperature vs. energy density factor. (Redrawn from Pearce, J.A., Geddes, L.A., Van Vleet, J., Foster, K., and Allen, J. *Med. Instrum.* 1983, 17: 225–231.)

at X is shown in Figure 18. Note that the return path is via the ECG monitoring electrodes, causing current to flow into the monitor and to any other contact between the patient and the grounded operating table, as shown by R at the patient's heel. Because these areas of contact are not large, the current density will be high and burns can result at these sites. Such alternate-path currents are by no means uncommon in accident cases.

BURNS UNDER ECG ELECTRODES

As just shown, if one or more of the ECG electrodes become part (or all) of the electrosurgical current path, skin burns can result. Wald (1971) reported such an incident; he stated:

> Throughout the surgical procedure the ECG trace on the cardioscope appeared normal, without excessive interference. At the end of the procedure when the ECG electrodes were removed, second-degree burns, approximately 0.5 × 0.5 cm in size, were noted under the right and left shoulder electrodes. ....Inspection of the cautery showed that one of the wires connecting the patient-plate to the cautery was broken.

Similar incidents were reported by Becker et al. (1974) when the ground electrode of the ECG acted as the return path for electrosurgical current because the wire to the dispersive electrode was broken.

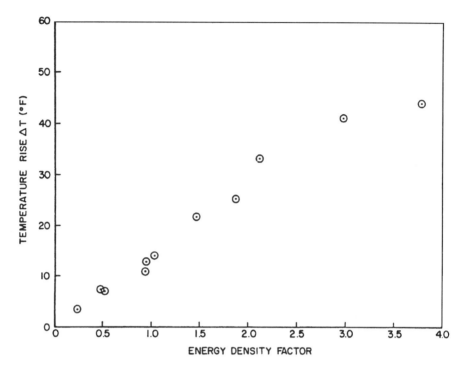

FIGURE 17 Skin-temperature rise under ECG-monitoring electrodes for different energy density factors. Calculated from DeRosa and Gadsby (1979).

A very common cause of skin burn results from inadequate contact between a dispersive electrode and the patient. Such a situation can arise after the electrode has been applied properly and the patient is repositioned, which can put a strain on the cable and partially remove the electrode. Repositioning a patient may cause the electrode to buckle, a situation known as "tenting". The author has investigated several cases in which there was inadequate contact with the patient after initial correct application of the dispersive electrode, followed by placing the legs in stirrups as is used in obstetrics and gynecology. In these cases, burns occurred at the dispersive electrode site.

TEMPERATURE -PROBE ACCIDENTS

Body temperature is measured frequently during anesthesia because anesthetic agents depress the body's temperature-regulating system. Therefore, the temperature of a patient in a cool operating room will decrease with the passage of time. Two sites, (1) rectum and (2) esophagus, are often used for placement of an electrical temperature probe. Injuries at these sites have been reported in association with the use of electrosurgery.

Wald (1971) reported a case of burn in the rectum of a patient in whom a battery-operated temperature probe had been installed. In describing the temperature-sensing system Wald stated:

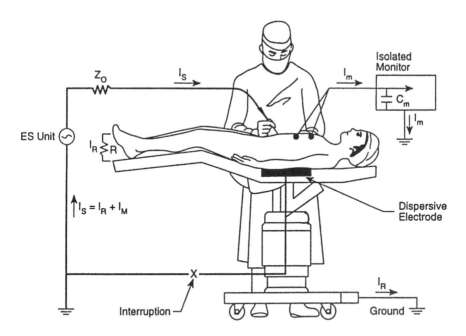

FIGURE 18   Alternate current paths when the dispersive electrode lead is interrupted. Leakage current (I_R) can flow from the body to the operating table and current (I_m) can flow into a patient monitor.

It is a battery-operated portable device consisting of a case which contains the electronic components and battery, and a probe which contains the temperature-sensing element at its tip. The telethermometer case is metal, but is finished all around with insulated surfaces. In addition, on the bottom surface of the case there are four short (0.5-mm) cork legs which are intended to keep the case electrically isolated from the surface on which it rests. Thus, in design, battery operation and case construction completely isolate the case from ground or any other electronic equipment. However, in practice, examination of several telethermometer cases has shown the insulated surfaces scratched in various areas, exposing the metal. Also, the cork feet can be worn or fall off, which brings the exposed surface of the case in contact with its support. In operating room use, the telethermometer case normally rests on a well-grounded pedestal.

The foregoing clearly shows that the temperature probe formed part of the return path for the electrosurgical current.

An esophageal burn at the site of a temperature probe was reported by Parker (1984). The patient underwent knee surgery and the electrosurgical dispersive electrode was placed on the left thigh. Parker reported:

The operation, lasting slightly over 4 h, was devoid of any unusual anesthetic or surgical events. There were no arrhythmias, and the esophageal temperature ranged between 35.5 and 35.9°C. However, the temperature probe, after removal, was noted to have several smooth dark brown and black areas of discoloration on the white surface not noted prior to its insertion. After a routine emergence and extubation of the trachea in the operating room, the patient was admitted to the recovery room in a drowsy, easily arousable, stable condition, with blood pressure 130/80 mmHg, heart rate 84 beats/min, and respiratory rate 20 breaths/min while receiving 40% humidified oxygen via face mask.

In recovery room, approximately 1 h after admission, the patient began spitting up copious amounts of blood-tinged saliva. Auscultation of the lungs revealed generalized congestion. An immediate chest radiograph revealed right hilar opacification. Vital signs remained stable with blood pressure 150/80 mmHg, heart rate 90 beats/min, and respiratory rate 20 breaths/min, without dyspnea or ectopy. An elective awake left nasotracheal intubation was performed because of increasing hemoptysis. Approximately 2 h later, copious amounts of frothy red sputum were suctioned. The patient breathed 10 1/min oxygen via a T-tube, arterial blood gases revealing a pH 7.27, PaO_2 302 mmHg, $PaCO_2$ 50.7 mmHg, and BE –4.4 mEq/l. A general surgeon then performed esophagoscopy and flexible bronchoscopy. Bronchoscopy revealed frothy, bloody fluid from the right main stem bronchus with the posterior tracheal wall blistered and red. Esophagoscopy revealed the probable site of primary burn as the middle of esophagus with whitened (linear) burns. The patient then was sedated, treated with steroids and antibiotics, and ventilation controlled. He made a rapid and uneventful recovery with no apparent permanent adverse sequele.

It was later found that the temperature probe was grounded. Despite its distance from the dispersive electrode on the left thigh, the temperature probe carried enough return-path electrosurgical current during the 4-h operation to produce the burn. The instruction manual for the temperature probe cautioned:

> In medical use, remove the probe from patient contact before activating electrosurgical apparatus or other direct-coupled RF energy source.

ENDOSCOPIC ELECTROSURGERY

New surgical techniques with endoscopes have introduced "minimally invasive surgery" and shortened in-hospital stays considerably. However, endoscopic electrosurgical techniques merit scrutiny for potential hazards because such endoscopes operate in cramped, electrically hostile environments. Although there are many types of endoscopic techniques, they may be classified as single-entry site or multiple-entry site techniques. The cystoscope or resectoscope (Figure 19) is an example of the former. Laparoscopy (Figure 20) uses two instruments and often two additional entry sites for holding instruments. The laparoscope is passed through a trocar into a body cavity. The trocar may be of metal or plastic. The endocsope may have many lumens; the model shown in Figure 20A contains a lumen for inflating the body cavity with a nonflammable gas, e.g., carbon dioxide. There is a lumen for a fiberoptic bundle which illuminates the cavity, and a lumen for a telescope for viewing the operating site; sometimes a video camera is mounted to the eyepiece and a video monitor displays the body cavity. Two additional trocars may be used for the passage of grasping tools. Figure 20 also shows a grasping forceps that is passed into the body cavity. The shaft of the forceps is electrically insulated and electrosurgical current

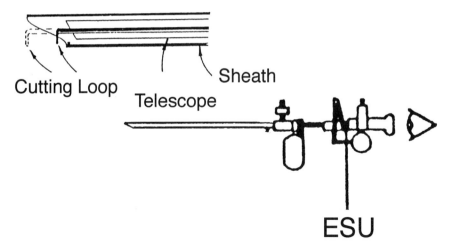

FIGURE 19 A resectoscope showing the cutting loop.

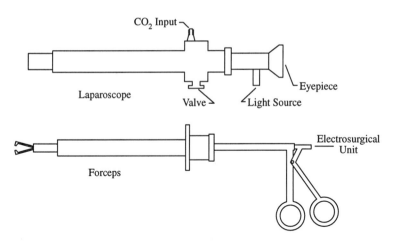

FIGURE 20 Endoscope and grasping forceps.

is applied to coagulate the tissue between the jaws. There are many other types of instruments used with endoscopes (e.g., scissors, loops, snares, etc.).

From an electrical viewpoint, there are several types of endoinstruments; one has an inner conductor that is insulated from the metal sheath and the other has an insulating covering over the metal shaft that carries the electrosurgical current. There are older instruments in which the metal shaft is uninsulated and the surgical gloves afford the only protection for the operator.

Figure 21 characterizes the situation when a sterilized forceps is inserted into a body opening or one made with a trocar. The metal sheath of the endoinstrument is insulated. A sterilized cable connects the instrument to the ESU. With the tip of the active electrode in contact with tissue, the ESU is activated and the solid arrow in

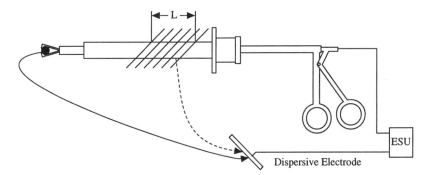

FIGURE 21 Grasping forceps with electrical insulation covering the metal parts and principal current path (solid arrow) and alternate current path (dashed arrow).

Figure 21 identifies the principal current path. Because of the insulation there is a distributed capacitance between the metal sheath of the forceps and the patient. Consequently, there is a current path to the surrounding tissue (via region L) to the dispersive electrode; this alternate current path is shown by the dashed arrow in Figure 21. If the distributed capacitance C = 100 pF, the reactance of C at 0.5 and 2 MHz is 3185 and 796 ohms, respectively. This means that in normal operation, the current in the alternate path is small. However, Hayes (1979) reported that with some instruments this alternate current amounts to 1/3 to 1/2 of the total current. If the forceps is uninsulated and passed through a plastic trocar, the current in the alternate path would be less. If the forceps were uninsulated and in contact with the body wall, the alternate current would be a substantial fraction of the total current.

Figure 22A illustrates schematically an endoinstrument in which a central current-carrying conductor is insulated from the metal sheath and the active electrode is not in contact with tissue and the ESU is activated. The dashed arrow identifies the current path. In this case the ESU (open-circuit) voltage would be high and the current due to the distributed capacitance (C) would be the major current path. Table 3 lists the open-circuit peak-to-peak voltage of typical ESUs for the different modes of use.

If the ESU output setting is high and the active electrode is not in contact with tissue, an arc could form between the active electrode and the metal sheath of the endoinstrument, as shown in Figure 22B, and a high current could flow from the sheath to the dispersive electrode. Such a situation could occur if the tip of the instrument is in a gas-filled cavity. Consequently, the instrument sheath resembles an active electrode and the patient and/or the operator could be burned. The burn will be severe if the area of contact of an uninsulated sheath with the patient is small.

The situation illustrated in Figure 22B is hazardous to the surgeon who is holding the endoscope with gloved hands. Because the voltage on the endoscope is high, there is the likelihood of breakdown of the insulation on the instrument and the gloves, resulting in a burn sustained by the patient and surgeon, a situation that is not unknown. The breakdown voltage for gloves was discussed earlier in this chapter.

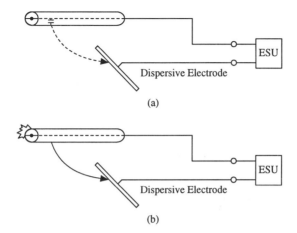

FIGURE 22   In (a) is shown an endoinstrument in which the current-carrying conductor is insulated from the metal sheath and the ESU is activated with the active electrode not in contact with the tissue. In (b) is shown an arc between the current-carrying conductor and metal sheath of the endoinstrument.

TABLE 3
Output Characteristics of Electrosurgical Units

	Output Voltage Range Open Circuit, $V_{peak-peak}$	Output Power Range, W
Monopolar Modes		
Cut	200–5,000	1–400
Blend	1,500–5,800	1–300
Desiccate	400–6,500	1–200
Fulgurate/spray	6,000–12,000	1–200
Bipolar Mode		
Coagulate/desiccate	400–100	1–70

Data from von Maltzahn and Eggelston. *Biomedical Engineering Handbook,* Bronzino, J., Ed. 1995. CRC Press, Boca Raton, FL.

UROLOGICAL APPLICATIONS

Electrosurgery is used extensively in urology; for example, it is used to increase the diameter of the urethra that has been narrowed by prostatic enlargement, the operation being known as transurethral resection (TUR). Other uses include the removal of tumors or polyps in the bladder. The current levels are the highest and the activation times are the longest in all of electrosurgery (see Table 1).

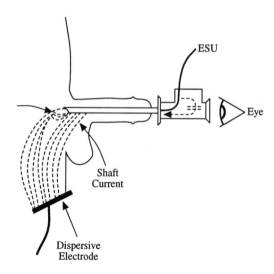

FIGURE 23 Current flow from the tip electrode and shaft of a cystoscope.

In bladder electrosurgery, the resectoscope is passed into the bladder via the urethra as shown in Figure 23. The bladder is first evacuated of its highly conducting urine and filled with a poorly conducting isotonic fluid, such as 5% dextrose in water. In this process, the operating area is usually quite wet, contributing to electrical hazard.

The shafts of some resectoscopes are bare metal; others are covered with a thin layer of electrical insulation. To improve current distribution Flachenecker and Fastenmeier (1979) recommended the use of a conducting lubricant if the resectoscope sheath is uninsulated and a poorly conducting lubricant if the resectoscope sheath is insulated.

In transurethral resection the cutting loop of the resectoscope (Figure 19) is advanced and withdrawn to ablate tissue to enlarge the urethra. Owing to the capacitance between the conductor carrying current to the loop and the metal sheath of the resectoscope there is current flow from the shaft to the patient, as shown in Figure 23.

Cutting loops can be bent or broken and come into contact with the metal sheath of the resectoscope, thereby making it an active electrode and presenting a hazard to the urologist and patient. Careful inspection of the resectoscope prior to sterilization is essential. The cable from the resectoscope to the ESU must be inspected carefully for continuity and insulation cracks before each sterilization. Cracks in insulation favor the genesis of a spark which could produce injury or be a source of ignition. Although steam sterilization is the best, it is hard on cables and insulation. Manufacturers of resectoscopes (and other endoinstruments) and cables provide recommendations for sterilization that must be followed to insure patient and operator safety.

In summary, among the hazards associated with urologic electrosurgery are burns due to accidental contact with tissues other than those intended, as well as those due to alternate current paths, muscle contraction, and interference with patient monitoring equipment and implanted electronic devices, such as cardiac pacemakers and automatic implanted cardioverter defibrillators (AICDs). The use of a temporary cardiac pacing lead with an external pacemaker in the vicinity of an ESU is hazardous and may result in ventricular fibrillation; these cases are discussed in the chapter on EMI. Because urologic electrosurgery uses the highest current levels and the longest activation times, the opportunity for accidents is high.

As discussed previously, leg muscle contraction frequently accompanies TUR procedures and arises from stimulation of the obturator nerve which courses near the prostate. Stimulation of this nerve by electrosurgical current causes the leg to move toward the midline. Hodika and Clarke (1961) advocated the use of myoneural blocking agents to abolish muscle contraction. However, the use of such agents also paralyzes the muscles of respiration and positive-pressure breathing must be applied.

INJURY TO THE UROLOGIST

Whereas most resectoscopic injuries are suffered by the patient, urologists have been injured while performing a transurethral resection. For example, Thomas (1975) reported that he was using:

An Iglesias resectoscope element with a telescope fitted with the photographic type eyepiece. The current supplying the resectoscope came from an electrosurgical unit of the spark-gap variety. During the operation the entire instrument heated and warmth emanated to the surgeon's hands. Various parts of the instrument were exchanged but the final instrument was as described. While cutting a piece of tissue the author experienced sudden severe pain in the right eye. The pain was so intense that the operation had to be completed by another surgeon. Examination by an ophthalmologist revealed a burn and laceration to the cornea. The eye was treated symptomatically and conservatively with the resulting residual effects of myopia and uniocolar diplopia producing 4 images in the injured eye.

After investigating the accident, Thomas reported:

Analysis of this accident revealed the photographic eyepiece as being responsible for allowing arcing to occur to the surgeon's eye. More specifically, the metal resectoscope post protruding through the center of the eyepiece allowed the arcing to occur. The investigation of this accident confined itself to the instrument being used. However, many eyepieces (in daily use) have metal exposed around the plano lens of the telescope ocular and are, in the opinion of this author, unsafe for use with electrosurgical units inasmuch as unrelated electrical problems or system breakdown exposes the surgeon's eyes to a risk of serious injury.

An accident investigated by the author resulted in a serious back injury to the urologist. The bladder had been emptied of urine and filled with D5W. The resectoscope was in place ready to perform a transuretheral resection. The urologist was looking through the eyepiece and activated the electrosurgical unit. Immediately he fell off his stool, bending the bracket on the operating table that held the drainage basin, and landed on the floor in extreme pain such that he could not get up. The anesthesiologist deadened the dorsal nerve roots to abolish the pain. The urologist

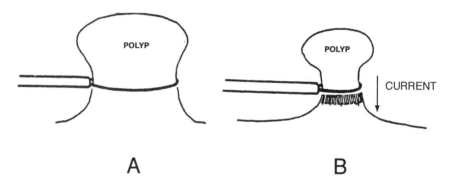

FIGURE 24   Snare around the stalk of a polyp (A) and electrosurgical current direction (B).

suffered so much injury to the spine that he could no longer perform many of the duties of a urologist.

On examination of the resectoscope and its cable, it was found that there was a break in the cable at the connector. On interrogating the urologist, he reported that an arc struck his nose when the ESU was activated and this shock caused him to lose his balance and fall. Note that with a broken cable, the ESU is operating under an open-circuit condition and the voltage is very high, favoring the production of an arc.

POLYPECTOMY

A polyp is a pedunculated growth arising from the mucosa and extending into the lumen of an organ. A polyp can be removed with the aid of a cystoscope, colonoscope, sigmoidoscope, or proctoscope. The procedure often employs a wire snare to which electrosurgical current is applied. Figure 24A illustrates the snare around the stalk and Figure 24B shows the direction of current flow down the stalk which is coagulated, then cut by the current. Alternately, the coagulated stalk can be cut mechanically by tightening the snare. Some surgeons use blended current to coagulate and cut the stalk.

In Figure 24B, the electrosurgical current flows down the stalk to the cavity wall. This situation will occur only if the top of the polyp is not contacting any other conducting tissue. If the top of the polyp is in contact with tissue, current will flow up the stalk and a burn may occur at the top contact site.

EXPLOSIONS IN THE GASTROINTESTINAL TRACT

It should be remembered that the gastrointestinal tract contains flammable gases: methane, hydrogen, and a small quantity of hydrogen sulfide; Table 4 shows the maximum and minimum values reported by Levy (1954). The average values should be noted in which there is 7.2% methane and 20.9% hydrogen with 3.9% oxygen. In his paper Levy discussed the proportions for combustion. The composition of bowel gas is influenced by the amount of milk and legumes ingested (Table 5). On the average diet, the bowel content for hydrogen is about 21% and for methane it

TABLE 4
Composition of Intestinal Gas

Intestinal Gas Found (%)	CO$_2$	O$_2$	CH$_4$	H$_2$	N$_2$
Highest...	25.4	20.0	44.0	43.9	87.0
Lowest...	00.0	00.0	00.0	00.0	24.7
Average	9.0	3.9	7.2	20.9	9.0
Volume of flatus average 1.48 ml/min					

Data from Levy, E.I. *Am. J. Surg.* 1954, 88: 754–758.

TABLE 5
Bowel Gas Composition

Diet	H$_2$ (%)	Methane (%)
Average	21	7
Milk	44	
Legume		44

is about 7%. On a milk diet, gut hydrogen increases to about 44%, and on a legume diet, methane also increases to about 44%. It should be recognized that the bowel contains oxygen from swallowed air. Therefore, an explosive mixture can be present. Ignition of these gases is easily accomplished by a spark from an active electrosurgical electrode. The ensuing explosion can produce a disastrous accident; the following are a few examples from the published literature which reveals a pre-existing knowledge of the hazard.

Arnous (1945) described an anoscope with which flowing carbon dioxide (2L/min) could be used during electrosurgery to avoid the hazard of bowel-gas explosion. Becker (1953) also advocated purging the bowel with carbon dioxide to prevent bowel-gas explosion. Woodward (1961) advocated passing carbon dioxide down the suction lumen of the endoscope. Hussey and Pois (1970) recommended "the use of a cold knife technique to open the bowel" before using electrosurgery. Apparently, these recommendations went unheeded because many bowel-gas explosions appeared in the subsequent literature.

Carter (1952) scheduled a patient for polypectomy and reported:

The patient was prepared with cleansing tap water enemas for sigmoidoscopic biopsy and electrodesiccation of the polyps. Without anesthesia the highest polyp was biopsied and its base destroyed by a desiccating current using a Birtcher Hyfrecator. The accumulated smoke was removed by suction and the sigmoidoscope was readjusted to bring the lower polyp into view. It was also biopsied and after the resulting blood in the bowel was evacuated with suction the desiccating current was applied to the base. An accumulation of smoke was removed from the bowel and the sigmoidoscope readjusted. It was noted that a small portion of the base of the polyp remained and the desiccating current was again applied to that area. When the current was turned on this last time, there was a sudden violent explosion within the bowel causing a blue flame to shoot out the end of the sigmoidoscope for a distance of one or two feet. A loud muffled sound that was audible into the adjoining room accompanied the explosion. The patient immediately screamed and started to climb off the examining table.

The patient was taken to the operating room for laparotomy. Carter continued:

There were numerous areas in the sigmoid colon which showed separation of the serosal coats of the bowel but with the mucous membrane intact. These areas were closed with interrupted sutures of No. 7-0 cotton. As the bowel was further examined it was found that the proximal one-half of the descending colon near the splenic flexure had been lacerated in many places and was actively bleeding. The lacerations measured up to 10 cm in length and involved all coats of the bowel. It was necessary to resect the distal end of the transverse colon, the splenic flexure and the proximal one-half of the descending colon in order to remove the lacerated portions of the bowel and to control bleeding. The ends of the colon were exteriorized at the superior and the inferior portions of the abdominal incision and two Penrose drains were placed in the peritoneal cavity.

Carter continued:

During his convalescent period he continued to complain of burning epigastric discomfort which had been present before the operation and on two or three occasions mild symptoms of partial intestinal obstruction developed which subsided with conservative management. Approximately three months following the accident the abdomen was reopened and after freeing numerous intestinal adhesions the two ends of the colon were anastomosed. Following the operation the patient's course was uneventful and he began to have normal bowel movements through his rectum on the fourth post-operative day.

The term "detonation" was used by Zimmerman (1959) to describe a bowel-gas explosion in a 79-year-old, 82-lb lady admitted for occasional bleeding at the stool. Zimmerman stated:

A proctoscopic examination showed moderate sized internal hemorrhoids and a sessile adenoma 0.5 cm in diameter on the anterior wall of the rectum at the 4 inch level. The patient complained so much during the examination that no treatment was attempted and no biopsy taken.

Five days later she consented to have the polyp removed. A plain water enema was given the night before, and repeated at 11 a.m. on the morning of the anticipated removal. There is no definite record of what she ate during the 24 h previous to this incident, but she had little appetite and had only picked at her food since her admission to the hospital.

At 2:30 p.m. she was placed in the invert position and a 7/8 by 8 in. sigmoidoscope inserted into her bowel. The adenoma was located without difficulty. A 10 in. electropoint, connected to the single pole of a Hyfrecator which was adjusted to its highest setting, was touched to the lesion. As the current was turned on by the foot-switch, there was a muffled but loud explosion. This noise was loud enough to be heard in the hall outside the room even though the door was closed.

The sigmoidoscope and electropoint were withdrawn reflexly at the time of the explosion, and the patient jumped up and screamed, "You tore me apart!" After a minute or two she was persuaded to lie back on the table, and the sigmoidoscope was reinserted. The rectum seemed a little pale, but otherwise showed no sign of damage. The mucous membrane of the sigmoid colon was torn in irregular ragged lines as might be expected from overstretching, and was bleeding. No perforations were seen. No pictures were taken at this time as a camera was not available. Examination of the abdomen showed it to be tense and tender. There was no discernible distention, and an occasional peristaltic gurgle could be heard. The pulse rate was 100. She was given 50 mg of meperidine (Demerol) intramuscularly. The blood was typed and cross-matched. She was sent for a plain X-ray film of the abdomen: this showed no free air in the abdominal cavity.

Careful medical management was applied and Zimmerman stated:

One week after the incident, another proctosigmoidoscopy was performed. The rectum appeared normal, while the sigmoid still contained some small white irregular areas of healing. The membrane between these patches was normal. Since discharge from the hospital, the patient has had no abdominal complaints. Her bowels are moving regularly without cathartics, but she refuses to come to the office for any further examination or treatment.

Zimmerman was aware that methane and hydrogen could be in the intestinal tract and that both were explosive. To eliminate the hazard, he recommended: "(1) to place the end of the instrument tightly against the mucous membrane surrounding the polyp, thereby isolating it; and (2) to force carbon dioxide across the area being treated."

A colostomy explosion was described by Bellemore (1962) in a patient who had a colonic lavage for three days prior to surgery and who was on a low-residue diet. After removing a tumor, a loop of transverse colon was brought to the abdominal wall to fashion a colostomy. Bellemore wrote:

After the paramedian incision was sealed, it was decided to open the colostomy with the [surgical] diathermy. A violent explosion occurred, a blast of air shot past my face and I thought that the patient had succumbed. However, the patient's condition was unchanged, but where the colon had been incised there was an irregular opening the size of a 2-shilling piece. After some deliberation it was decided not to reopen the abdomen although it was realized that the caecum probably had borne the brunt of the explosion. I regretted this decision later and in retrospect it was an error of judgment.

Her condition remained unchanged for some 4 to 6 h and then it was apparent that the blast had produced serious damage. There was profuse sero-sanguinous discharge from the drainage tube and the patient's systolic blood pressure fluctuated between 70 and 90 mm of mercury. Blood and later several bottles of serum albumen were administered as the profuse serous drainage continued. Within 48 h fluid faeces were draining through the tube and gradually the patient's general condition improved.

It is obvious that there were explosive gases in the colon and that entry into it to open the colostomy using an active electrosurgical electrode provided the igniting spark.

An explosion associated with cauterization of a large polyp in the rectum was reported by Ross (1961), who wrote:

> The first, second, and third cauterizations were administered without incident. However, during the fourth session, with the patient in the genupectoral position and the proctoscope inserted about 5 cm cauterization was begun. After about three minutes there was an explosion within the bowel. The impact of the explosion was so violent that the proctoscope and the cautery were blown out of the rectum, landing a considerable distance from the operating table.
>
> Two linear perforations were discovered on the border of the sigmoid flexure opposite the mesenteric attachment. Each perforation was 2 cm long, loops of small intestine were dilated and a small quantity of dark fluid had accumulated in the cul-de-sac of Douglas. The splits in the intestine were closed in two layers and a provisional colostomy was established. The postoperative period was uneventful.

In the foregoing case, the intestinal tract was not purged of gases, probably because the polyp was so near the anus. It is likely that the explosion resulted from propulsion of intestinal gas by peristalsis during the surgical procedure.

Another explosion was reported by Bigard et al. (1979). The patient was admitted for the removal of a cecal polyp. The patient preparation included a 2-day, nonresidue diet and an intestinal lavage (5 l of isotonic solution) the evening before the operation. They reported:

> After locating the polyp, it was snared with an Olympus diathermy snare connected to the Olympus PSD electrosurgical source. No inert gas was insufflated. A coagulating current was used, the control being on setting 4. After 8–10 sec of current passage, there was an explosion which was audible in the endoscopy room, the patient jerked upwards off the endoscopy table, and the colonoscope was completely ejected. The diathermy snare contained only a small portion of the polyp.
>
> The patient immediately showed clinical signs of shock and complained of generalized abdominal pain. Examination showed evidence of massive pneumoperitoneum with a distended abdomen and loss of hepatic dullness to percussion. Needle puncture of the abdomen released a large quantity of gas and slightly reduced the abdominal pain. The patient was immediately transferred to the operating theater, and laparotomy was carried out 15 min after explosion. Immediately on opening the abdomen a hemoperitoneum was visible. There was no fecal matter in the abdomen. Examination of the colon showed numerous full-thickness lacerations in the right colon and the transverse colon as far as the splenic flexure. There were multiple bleeding points around these perforations. In addition the spleen was found to have numerous capsular lacerations. An extended right hemicoloectomy was carried out to include the right colon, the transverse colon, and the splenic flexure. Massive blood transfusion was continued during the whole procedure; the patient received 45 units of blood. Multiple bleeding points occurred in all areas of dissection (right flank, left hypochondrium, and the pancreatic region), and it proved impossible to achieve hemostasis. There was presumably a serious coagulation defect as a result

of the multiple transfusions, and the surgeon closed the abdomen after packing the abdomen. Death occurred a few minutes later.

Barkman (1965) reported another bowel-gas explosion in a patient who was admitted for resection of a carcinoma of the rectosigmoid colon. He wrote:

The caecum was then opened, using the cutting [surgical] diathermy. Some sparking took place at the point of the diathermy needle on cutting through the caecal wall, and immediately the point entered the lumen of the bowel a loud explosion took place with a forcible upward rush of gas and a small amount of faeces. The noise of the explosion was considerable, but no flash or burning was noted by any of the attendants at the operation. A few seconds later, however, a small puff of white smoke was noted coming from the drainage-tube in the left iliac fossa.

The report was followed by an immediate fall in the patient's blood-pressure to 110/60 mm Hg from 140/100 mm Hg, which was the level during the operation, and the pulse rate dropped to 65, with poor volume. The operating table was tipped into the Trendelenburg position, and within 15 minutes the blood-pressure settled back at the level it had maintained during the operation. The pulse rate became steady at 70, with good volume. No signs of burning were noted at the site of the explosion or the surrounding skin. No inflammatory gases were in use by the anesthetist at the time of the explosion, nor, indeed, had any been used at any time throughout the operation.

The patient's abdomen was carefully examined after the explosion by several people and nothing untoward could be detected clinically, but the problem of deciding, at that time, whether there had been any visceral damage was a difficult one. As her general condition had recovered so well in a short time it was decided that no good purpose would be served by immediate re-exploration of the abdomen. The caecostomy was therefore sutured to the skin and a catheter inserted into the bowel lumen through the caecostomy.

After a further period of observation in the theatre with maintenance of her satisfactory general condition, she was returned to the ward and kept under close observation.

Her general condition started to deteriorate in the late afternoon of the day of operation, as evidenced by a progressive fall in blood pressure and rise in pulse rate, and it became increasingly difficult to maintain her blood pressure by various resuscitative measures.

In spite of vigorous resuscitative measures it was found impossible to maintain her blood pressure, and she died some 30 h after operation.

Commenting on the post-mortem findings, Barkman wrote:

The caecum and ascending colon were comparatively normal in appearance, which is interesting, as the explosion initiated in the caecum. Several large perforations were present in the colon, particularly in the hepatic and splenic flexures. There was evidence of early abscess formation in the region of the hepatic flexure. The small bowel and the other viscera appeared to be unaffected by the blast.

A stomach explosion was reported by Carroll (1964) who wrote:

There was a hard mass 2 in. (5 cm) in diameter obstructing the duodenum. It was decided to open the stomach and empty it and then perform a gastrojejunostomy. Diathermy was used and an opening made in the stomach wall; as soon as the mucosa was incised a loud explosion occurred which was heard outside the operating theatre. The escaping gases had ignited and were burning with an intense blue flame, but with no odour. An attempt was made to extinguish the flame with swabs, but after about 10 seconds it had ceased. At the same time the anaesthetist, thinking that the explosion might have been due to anaesthetic gases, quickly wheeled his trolley out of the theatre. In retrospect, the explosion could not have been caused by the gases he was using (oxygen, nitrous oxide, and halothane, with intermittent suxamethonium chloride). The stomach was then emptied and a gastrojejunostomy performed. The patient made an uneventful recovery.

LAPAROSCOPIC STERILIZATION

Since the early 1970s, the laparoscope has been used in conjunction with electro-surgery for sterilization by coagulating the Fallopian tubes. Typically, a monopolar grasping forceps is used to which electrosurgical current is applied. Sometimes the more preferable and safer bipolar technique is employed.

With the monopolar technique (Figure 25), the grasping forceps fitted with a biopsy sleeve is used. A fallopian tube is grasped and fulguration current is applied to the forceps to coagulate the tube. When a sufficient length of tube is coagulated, the rotary biopsy sleeve is advanced to cut off the coagulated tissue. The biopsy sleeve may not be used by some operators.

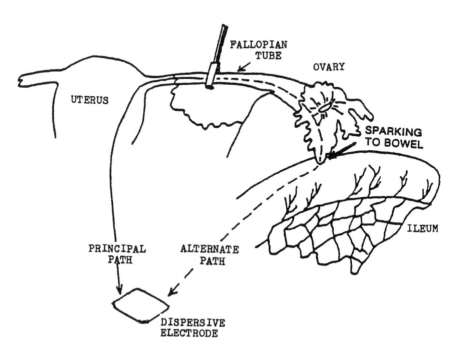

FIGURE 25 Tubal sterilization with electrosurgical current applied to a grasping forceps.

Basically, two types of injury have been supported with the endoscope: (1) injury at the site of entry when a metal trocar is used and (2) perforation of the bowel due to sparking. The following cases illustrate these injuries.

Referring to Figure 25, note that the principal current path (solid arrow) is from the monopolar forceps, along the fallopian tube to the uterus, and thence through the body to the dispersive electrode. However, there is an alternate current path (dashed arrow) along the fallopian tube to the ovary and thence to the ileum. Sparking and small-bowel perforation have been reported. A potentially hazardous situation arises if multiple regions of the fallopian tube are coagulated; the hazard depends on the order in which the coagulated regions are created. Coagulated tissue becomes a poor conductor of electric current; therefore, to minimize current flow to the ovary and sparking to the ileum, the first coagulation should be made closer to the ovary; the second and subsequent coagulations should be made advancing toward the uterus along the fallopian tube. In this way after the first coagulation, the principal current path is along the tube toward the uterus.

Tubal Coagulation Accidents

A variety of unusual accidents have accompanied tubal coagulation. For example, Esposito (1973) reported an abdominal wall burn due to a metal trocar used in conjunction with a grasping forceps. He reported on a 30-year-old female who was transferred from the emergency room because of pain in the lower abdomen. He reported:

She had laparoscopy and tubal cautery on March 23, 1972. At the time of tubal cautery, an area of hyperemia, approximately 3 cm, had been noted around the lateral trocar sleeve. Her postoperative course was, however, unremarkable and she was discharged on March 24, 1972.

She presented in the Emergency Room on March 27, 1972, complaining of pain in the lower abdomen of 1-day duration. Temperature, 102.4°; blood pressure, 110/70; pulse, 104. Physical examination was unremarkable except for the abdominal findings: an area of necrosis approximately 4 cm with a silk stitch in the center was noted. This was surrounded by a zone of hyperemia of approximately 2 cm. This portion of the abdomen was markedly tender. The rest of the abdomen was tender but soft. Bowel sounds were hypoactive. She was allowed nothing by mouth and Ampicillin was administered intravenously.

The patient was taken to the Operating Room on March 28, 1972, at 3:30 p.m. Exploration was performed through a midline incision and the intestines were found intact. The peritoneal surface under the burn was examined and did not appear to have been damaged. The abdomen was closed, the burnt skin and subcutaneous tissue were excised down to the fascia, and a culture was taken. The fascia was intact and did not show signs of thermal damage.

Postoperatively, the antibiotic was changed to Keflin, by mouth, and her temperature returned to normal on March 30, 1972. The wound was healing well when the patient was discharged on April 2, 1972. She was followed in the Surgical Clinic until complete healing.

In the case under discussion, we believe that the metal trocar sleeve must have come in contact with the conductive portion of the coagulating forceps. The trocar then conducted current from the tip of the forceps to the peritoneum, muscle fascia, subcutaneous tissue, and skin. The depth of the injury must have been directly proportional to the amount of current, the sensitivity of the tissues involved, and the time of exposure.

To assist future users of laparoscopic electrosurgery for sterilization, Esposito made three recommendations: (1) use a nonconducting trocar, (2) use minimal electrosurgical current, and (3) if a conductive sleeve is used, it must not contact the grasping forceps.

Levinson et al. (1973) reported that a 24-year-old female patient underwent bilateral tubal coagulation on October 5, 1971 without incident. She later reported:

On Oct. 8, 1971 the patient was readmitted to the hospital after a sudden onset of lower abdominal pain that became increasingly severe within 30 minutes. In the lower abdomen, there was marked guarding, marked tenderness on palpation and rebound tenderness. No definitive pelvic masses were determined, but there was marked paracervical tenderness.

The patient was taken to surgery the evening of October 8, 1971, with a differential diagnosis of small bowel perforation secondary to cautery vs. pelvic inflammatory disease. There was no evidence of acute inflammatory disease and the site of the tubal cauterization appeared to be normal for this stage of postoperative recovery. In the proximal ileum, an area of perforation with localized coagulation necrosis was identified. An area of approximately 2 cm surrounding the perforation appeared to represent burned tissue. Therefore, it was elected to resect a 3- to 4-inch segment of small intestine.

Levinson et al. (1973) reported a second case of a 23-year-old-female who underwent laparoscopic tubal coagulation on December 3, 1971, with the patient experiencing an uneventful recovery. They then stated:

She was readmitted to the hospital after she developed sudden lower abdominal pain. Diffuse abdominal tenderness with moderate distention of the lower abdomen was noted. The tenderness was most marked in the right lower quadrant. On pelvic examination, no abnormalities were noted. A culdocentesis revealed 10 ml straw-colored fluid. The patient was treated conservatively for several days. On December 13, 1971, exploratory laparotomy revealed perforation of the distal ileum with a localized area of necrosis. Approximately 6 inches of ileum was resected.

In discussing the cases, they stated that the ESU had not been inadvertently activated. They stated that "there was no evidence of direct coagulation, sparking probably occurred with a focal point of injury to the adjacent viscera."

Schwimmer (1974) reported three cases of small-bowel burn associated with laparoscopic tubal coagulation. One additional case provides evidence of a burn at the site of the trocar. He wrote:

When the instruments were removed, a burn was seen at the trocar site involving the skin, subcutaneous fat, fascia, muscle, and peritoneum. The central area was firm and white, and surrounded by a thin margin of pink tissue. A 3 × 5-cm ellipse of skin was excised together with all of the subcutaneous tissue and fascia that appeared nonviable, but the coagulated muscle was not removed. On the second postoperative day, the wound was slightly tender. By the fourth postoperative day it was no longer tender but there was a serosanguineous discharge. The patient had remained afebrile and was discharged to be followed as an outpatient. One week later, the area became erythematous and mild fever developed, which promptly subsided in response to a 10-day course of ampicillin. Complete healing required 6 to 7 weeks.

An unusual peritoneal explosion occurred during laparoscopic sterilization using electrosurgical current. El Kady and Abd-El-Razek (1976) reported:

Pneumoperitoneum was created using nitrous oxide gas introduced from a Boyle's anesthetic machine for 10 minutes (from induction of pneumoperitoneum to completion of electrocoagulation of both tubes at two sites). A final check via the laparoscope showed no bleeding nor any apparent damage to adjacent internal organs.

Immediately before withdrawing the Palmer forceps and the laparoscope, a loud explosion was heard. The laparoscope was broken into two parts. The upper part, nearly one-third of its length, was separated and blown away from the patient. The lower part of the laparoscope, still in the trocar, remained in the peritoneal cavity. The Palmer biopsy forceps was blown out of the peritoneal cavity. The puncture site was a ragged opening 2–3 cm in diameter. An immediate laparotomy was performed. All abdominal viscera were intact. The abdominal blood vessels appeared uninjured, and there was no intraperitoneal bleeding. A large tear at the center of the diaphragm, wide enough to admit a closed fist, was noted. A thoracotomy revealed that the heart was ruptured. The patient had died immediately.

The foregoing event occurred early in the development of this technique. Note that nitrous oxide, which is a noninflammable gas at room temperature, was used to inflate the peritoneal cavity. There was considerable speculation about its role in the accident. It is useful to note that above 300°C, nitrous oxide becomes a strong oxidizing agent. Many possible reasons for the accident were postulated, perhaps an unrecognized bowel perforation occurred with leakage of explosive gases into the peritoneal cavity.

Small bowel perforation was reported by Stewart et al. (1973) in a patient 10 days after laparoscopic sterilization. They stated:

At laparotomy, two areas of ulceration were seen on the antimesenteric surface of the ileum, 15 and 30 cm proximal to the ileocecal junction, which measured 1.5 by 2.5 cm. One of these had perforated. The lesions were excised, and the ileal wall was reconstituted, the patient thereafter making an uneventful postoperative recovery. Histologic examination of the excised tissue showed full-thickness necrosis of both lesions.

There being no evidence of other disease, the bowel wall injuries were considered to date from the time of sterilization. The cause of the damage however was not clear. Direct [surgical] diathermy burn due to contact of the diathermy forceps or forceps cannula against the bowel wall had not been suspected at operation. It was suggested that thermal injury to the bowel might have resulted from direct contact with the hot Fallopian tube closely following diathermy.

Several temperature-measurement experiments were carried out subsequently to determine if contact with the hot Fallopian tube could be implicated. Commenting on the experiments Stewart et al. stated:

The evidence derived from the above observations establishes that, although the tubal temperature of the point of diathermy is high, cooling occurs rapidly. Furthermore, attempts to produce damage to both parietal peritoneum and appendix wall when these structures were held against the hot Fallopian tube resulted in only trivial lesions.

They concluded:

It would appear, therefore, that the lesions described in the introductory case were unlikely to have been caused as a result of contact with the recently diathermized Fallopian tubes. (The issue of possible sparking to the bowel was not discussed.)

Peterson et al. (1981) reported another case of bowel injury associated with laparoscopic tubal sterilization; they wrote:

A healthy, 41-year-old woman, gravida 6, para 5, abortus 1, underwent laparoscopic tubal sterilization via electrocoagulation with a segment of each tube performed without apparent incident. The patient was discharged the day after operation.

Twenty-three days later, she returned to the hospital with abdominal pain and evidence of peritonitis. She gave a history of having been constipated for several days prior to admission but of otherwise doing well until shortly before entering the hospital, when she had begun to vomit and experience severe abdominal pain. When seen in the emergency room, the patient was found to be in septic shock.

The following morning, she underwent laparotomy. Purulent material was noted throughout the peritoneal cavity. Although the upper gastrointestinal tract was normal, the small and large bowels were covered by a large fibrinous exudate. Multiple adhesions were present and a perforation was noted on the anterior wall of the midportion of the sigmoid colon. A colectomy and diverting colostomy were performed. Histologic review of the 5 cm colectomy specimen revealed that the perforation had occurred at the site of a thermal injury. The patient's condition deteriorated and she died 41 days after laparotomy. Autopsy revealed a right-sided subdiaphragmatic abscess, peritonitis, and a small bowel perforation communicating with a subcutaneous abscess and fistula tract to the skin.

Peterson (1981) reported a second case as follows:

A healthy, 22-year-old woman, gravida 4, para 4, underwent dilatation and curettage followed by laparoscopic coagulation tubal sterilization with a unipolar device. The curettage proceeded without incident and yielded a scant amount of normal-appearing tissue. Electrocoagulation with resection and division of each fallopian tube was performed without apparent difficulty. The woman was discharged on the following day.

Seven days after the operation, the patient was hospitalized because of abdominal pain. She was febrile and had evidence of intestinal obstruction. Antibiotics were initiated, and an emergency laparotomy was performed. Findings included diffuse peritonitis. Although the surgeon believed preoperatively that bowel perforation had occurred, an attempt to identify the perforation site was unsuccessful. The effort was hampered because the bowel was covered with purulent material. No gastroduodenal perforation could be identified and the pelvis appeared entirely normal. Material from the abdominal cavity was cultured, the cavity was irrigated, and then the wound was closed.

After operation, the patient's condition deteriorated and she died 2 days later of septic shock. An autopsy was performed the following day. There were no new findings from those identified at surgery, i.e., no source of the peritonitis could be determined. Cultures of the abdominal cavity material grew *Enteribacter cloacae, Citrobacter freundii, Escherichia coli, Klebsiella pneumoniae, Clostridium perfringens,* and *Bacteroides* spp.

In commenting on these two cases, Peterson et al. concluded that thermal injury was sustained by the bowel in the first case and that perforation of the bowel occurred in the second case. This view was supported by the profuse purulent discharge covering the bowel and the growth of fecal flora in the cultures from the peritoneal cavity. They speculated on accidental contact of the bowel by the forceps and sparking. The foregoing injuries are not inconsistent with the alternate current path shown in Figure 25. Peterson et al. recommended the use of bipolar forceps.

The incidence of small-bowel perforations associated with laparoscopic tubal coagulation is small. For example, Thompson and Wheeless (1973) reported 10 such incidents in 3600 cases, providing an incidence of 0.28%. In a series of 7466 cases, Maudsley and Quizilbash (1979) reported only 4 small-bowel perforations, providing an incidence of 0.05%. In these four patients, symptoms of abdominal pain and tenderness appeared between 4 and 11 days. In all cases the lesions were sutured with the aid of the laparoscope and all patients survived.

CIRCUMCISION ACCIDENTS

Circumcision, the removal of all or part of the foreskin, is an ancient custom. Genesis 17: 10 states "Every male among you shall be circumcised." According to Gendron (1988), although circumcision is common in the U.S., it is uncomon in Great Britain and Australia. According to Gee and Ansell (1976), circumcision in the neonate is the second most frequently performed surgical procedure on the male in the U.S. They stated that controlling the small amount of bleeding presents no problem and the use of electrosurgery for this purpose is not recommended, especially when a metal clamp is used. Bloom et al. (1992) described circumcision as follows: "The skin is incised by knife or scissor (never with electrocautery when a metallic clamp is adjacent to the glans) and the clamp is left in place a full 10 min. The clamp is removed and the result is assessed to assure complete disruption of the adhesions and adequacy of the circumcision."

That a disastrous consequence can result when monopolar electrosurgery was used in association with circumcision in which a metal clamp was used was reported by Gee and Ansell (1976) who wrote:

Slough of the penis following Gomco circumcision in conjunction with the electro-surgical unit occurred at another hospital and is included because of the devastating result. A 4-month-old was circumcised electively in the operating room under anes-thesia; a Gomco device was used, and the surgeon employed the cutting current of an electrosurgical unit to excise the foreskin. Within five days, the glans and most of the shaft of the penis had sloughed. The patient was referred to this institution. Suprapubic cystostomy was done, and the patient underwent a number of staged procedures over two years to reconstruct the penis. These were unsuccessful, and the patient was surgically changed to a female.

An explanation for this tragic event is that the return path for all of the electro-surgical current was through the small-diameter, high-resistance penile shaft, result-ing in current crowding (Figure 13B) and thermal injury to this organ. When a monopolar electrode is used conventionally, the current spreads radially from the tip of the active electrode and tissue heating is confined to the tip area (see Figure 13A).

Another circumcision accident was reported by Strimling (1996), who used a Mogen clamp which fits over the glans. The case report stated:

This 3450-g term infant underwent circumcision with a Mogen clamp on his first day of life at his parent's request. His genital anatomy was notable only in that he had a relatively small penis, a scrotum that inserted about halfway up the penile shaft, and a considerable but not abnormal amount of redundancy of his foreskin.

The procedure was performed by a pediatrician who had extensive experience with this operation. The report continued:

Following a dorsal penile nerve block, the Mogen clamp was applied in the usual manner. When the clamp was removed it was obvious that the distal 2 mm (or tip) of the penis, including the urethral opening, had been amputated. This was imme-diately retrieved along with the foreskin remnant and placed in a medicine cup containing 10 ml of saline, which was then placed on ice.

With assistance of a plastic surgeon, the severed tip was reattached using micro-surgical techniques. Two years later, there was minimal cosmetic defect and normal urethral function. In discussing the case, Strimling stated:

Although circumcision with a Mogen clamp has been reported as easy, quick, and safe and is being taught in a number of centers, it may be that some children, particularly those with smaller organs or those with redundant foreskin, should not be considered as candidates for the use of this device. Although this may be an isolated event, as there is a reluctance to report adverse occurrences, the true risks of this device are not known.

SPERMATIC CORD COAGULATION

The author investigated an accident in which the spermatic cord of a neonate was coagulated. While performing the surgical repair of a hernia, the surgeon lifted a testis from the body and proceeded to trim tissue from the testis with monopolar electrode. When he looked down, the spermatic cord was coagulated and brownish in color. In this case, all of the electrosurgical current was carried by the slender cord, being an excellent example of current crowding or channeling.

Mitchell and Lumb (1966) and Schellhammer 1966) commented on such accidents. Schellhammer stated:

> Similar vessel damage may occur to penile vessels during circumcision or hypospadias' repair. Only later may testicular atrophy or distal penile necrosis be recognized.

He continued:

> If a saline-soaked sponge is placed under the cord and testes or penis, wide area contact with the thigh will prevent current channeling. Low generator voltage settings are advisable as well. The fact that heat concentration depends on the tissue volume interposed between electrodes makes it mandatory to reduce generator power for use in children because of the reduced size and volume of their structures.

NONELECTROSURGICAL SKIN INJURY

Some surgical procedures require a long time and a patient is rarely repostured. Despite the fact that a patient is lying on a padded surface, there arise regions of support where capillary perfusion is impaired. If there are sites where the pressure exceeds about 30 mmHg, the blood flow through capillaries at such sites is impaired, and if this situation lasts long enough, local tissue injury and death (necrosis) occur, resulting in what is known as bedsores or pressure sores. Various types of pressure mapping devices have been created (see Babbs et al., 1990) to identify the high-pressure sites in subjects lying on sleep surfaces. This subject is discussed in the chapter on skin injury. A good review of pressure sores was presented by Gendron (1988).

CONCLUSION

Electrosurgery achieves its goal by the controlled delivery of thermal energy at a desired site. With a monopolar electrode, the desired site is at the tip of the active electrode and nowhere else in the electrosurgical circuit. With a bipolar electrode, the desired site is between the tips of the bipolar electrode. The amount of thermal energy, and hence the heating, depends on the current density (squared) and the duration of activation (energy density factor). The heating is therefore maximum at the small-area electrode. The foregoing are the basic facts of electrosurgery and should be recognized by all who use it.

Particularly lacking by most in this field is an appreciation for the nature of radiofrequency (rf) current as it is used in electrosurgery. Such information can be found in the instruction manuals that accompany every ESU. Not only do these manuals discuss the various types of electrosurgical current, they also describe good electrosurgical technique and even illustrate hazardous situations. All who use electrosurgery should be required to prove that they have read the manual. There can be no doubt that the accident incidence can be decreased with better training and education. A starting point is to read the instruction manual.

It is useful to recognize that both old and new electrosurgical instruments are in daily use. The old spark-gap and vacuum-tube units have a long life and, for this reason, still see service. Therefore, when investigating an accident, the characteristics of the ESU must be determined.

Because of the nature of electrosurgical current, it is likely that it will continue to interfere with implanted electronic devices and environmental monitoring and therapeutic devices unless they are designed for immunity (hardened). Implanted devices, such as cardiac pacemakers and automatic defibrillators, can be adversely affected by the ESU, particularly if the electrosurgical current traverses electrodes connected to them. Care must be exercised in placing the dispersive electrode so that the return current path avoids such implants. Environmental monitoring devices can be improved to reduce their susceptibility to the ESU, or at least to recover quickly after cessation of electrosurgical current. It should be possible to render such external environmental devices as ventilators, drug-infusion pumps, etc. virtually immune from ESU current; however, such immunity has not been achieved yet.

Despite all of the hazards and accidents described in this chapter, their incidence is very small in comparison to the huge number of electrosurgeries performed annually. Perhaps the best method of reducing the number of accidents is via education programs for nurses and surgeons. All should be required to prove that they have read the instruction manual and should receive hazard training from the clinical engineer.

REFERENCES

AAMI (Association for the Advancement of Medical Instrumentation). 3330 Washington Blvd., Arlington, VA 22201-4598. AAMI Order Code HF18-R-2/93. Proposed 2nd edition of the *American National Standard for Electrosurgical Devices.*

American College of Surgeons. Conference on electrosurgery. *Surg. Gynecol. Obstet.* 1931, 52: 502–520.

Arnous, M.J. Anuscope permettant les electro-coagulations intra-rectales sous une atmosphere de gaz inerte. *Arch. d. mal. de l'app. digestif.* 1945, 34: 277–279.

Babbs, C.F., Bourland, J.D., Graber, G., et al. A pressure-sensitive mat for measuring contract pressure distribution of patients lying on hospital beds. *Med. Instr. Technol.*, 1990, 24: 363–370.

Barkman, M.F. Intestinal explosion after opening a caecostomy with diathermy. *Br. Med. J.* 1965, June: 1594–1595.

Becker, C.M., Malhotra, I.V., and Hedley-White, J. The distribution of radiofrequency current and burns. *Anesthesiology* 1974, 38(2): 106–122.

Becker, G.L. Prevention of gas explosions in the large bowel during electrosurgery. *Surg. Gynecd. Obst.*, 1953, 97: 463–467.

Bellemore, C. Colostomy explosion. *Austral. New Zealand J. Surg.* 1962, 31: 325–326.

Bigard, M.A., Gaucher, P., and Lassalle, C. Fatal colonic explosion during colonoscopic polypectomy. *Gastroenterology* 1979, 77: 1307–1310.

Bloom, D.A., Wan, J., and Key, D. Diseases of the male external genitalia and inguinal canal. In *Clinical Pediatric Urology.* Vol. 2, 3rd ed. 1992. W.B. Saunders, Philadelphia.

Carroll, K.J. Unusual explosion during electrosurgery. *Br.Med.J.* 1964, November: 78.

Carter, H.G. Explosion in the colon during electrodesiccation of polyps. *Am. J. Surg.* 1952, November: 514–517.

Caruso, P., Pearce, J.A., and DeWitt, D.P. Temperature and current density distributions at electrosurgical dispersive electrode sites. *Proc. 7th N. Engl. Bioeng. Conf.* 1979, 373–374.

Clark, W.L. Oscillatory desiccation in the treatment of accessible growths and minor surgical conditions. *J. Adv. Ther.* 1911, 29: 169–183.

Cushing, H. and Bovie, W.T. Electro-surgery as an aid to the removal of intracranial tumors. *Surg. Gynec. Obst.* 1928, 47: 751–784.

DeRosa, J. and Gadsby, P.D. Radiofrequency heating under ECG electrodes. *Med. Instrum.* 1979, 13: 273–276.

Doyen, E. Sur la destruction des tumeurs cancereuses accessible. *Arch. Elect. Med. Physiol.* 1909, 17: 791–795.

Doyen, E. *Surgical Therapeutics and Operative Techniques.* Vol. 1. 1917. William Wood, New York, 439-52.

El Kady, A.A. and Abd-El-Razek, M. Intraperitoneal explosion during female sterilization by laparoscopic electrocoagulation. *Int. J. Gynecol. Obst.* 1976, 14: 487–488.

Ellis, J.D. The rate of healing of electrosurgical wounds. *J.A.M.A.* 1931, 96: (1): 16–18.

Esposito, J.M. Electrical burn of the abdominal wall as a complication of Fallopian tube cautery. *Fertility Sterility* 1973, 24(2): 158–161.

Finlay, B., Couchie, D., Boyce, L., et al. Electrosurgery burns resulting from use of miniature ECG electrodes. *Anesthesiology* 1974, 41(3): 263–269.

Flachenecker, G. and Fastenmeier, K. High frequency current effects during transurethral resection. *J. Urol.* 1979, 122: 336–347.

Foster, K.S. and Geddes, L.A. The cause of stimulation with electrosurgical current. *Med. Instrum.* 1986, 20(6): 335–336.

Geddes, L.A., Silva, L.F., DeWitt, D.P., and Pearce, J.A. What's new in electrosurgical instrumentation. *Med. Instr.* 1977, 11(6): 385–389.

Geddes, L.A., Pearce, J.A., Bourland, J.D., et al. The thermal properties of gelled and metal-foil electrosurgical dispersive electrodes. *Proc. 14th AAMI Conf.*, 1979, 14: 90.

Geddes, L.A., Pearce, J.A., Bourland, J.D., and Silva, L.F. Thermal properties of dry metal-foil dispersive electrodes. *Clin. Eng.* 1980, 5: 13–18.

Geddes, L.A. and Moore, C. Stimulation with electrosurgical current. *Physics Eng. Sci. Med.* 1990, 13(2): 63–66 (Australia).

Gee, W.F. and Ansell, J.S. Neonatal circumcision. *Pediatrics* 1976, 58(6): 824–827.

Gendron, F.G. Unexplained Patient Burns. Quest Publishing, Brea, CA. 1988.

Hayes, C. Making laparoscopy electrically safer. *J. Reproductive Med.* 1979, 23(2): 92–93.

Hodika, J.H. and Clarke, G. Use of neuromuscular blocking drugs to counteract thigh adductor spasm induced by electrical shocks of obturator nerve during transurethral resection of bladder tumors. *J. Urol.* 1961, 85(3): 295–296.

Honig, W.M. The mechanism of cutting in electrosurgery. *IEEE Trans. BME* 1975, January: 60–62.

Hussey, G.L. and Pois, A.J. Bowel-gas explosion. *Am. J. Surg.* 1970, 120: 103–105.

Kelly, H.A. and Ward, G.E. *Electrosurgery.* 1932. W.B. Saunders, Philadelphia, 305.

Levinson, C.J., Schwartz, S.F., and Saltzstein, E.D. Complication of laparoscopic cauterization small bowel perforation. *Obst. Gynecol.* 1973, 41(2): 253–256.

Levy, E.I. Explosions during lower bowel electrosurgery. *Am. J. Surg.* 1954, 88: 754–758.

Maudsley, R.F. and Quizilbash, A.H. Thermal injury to the bowel as a complication of laparoscopic sterilization. *Can. J. Surg.* 1979, 22(3): 232–234.

McGreevy, F.T. and Bertrand, C. Electrosurgical Conductive Gas Stream Technique of Achieving Improved Eschar for Coagulation. U.S. Patent 4,781,175, November 1, 1988.

Mitchell, J.P. and Lumb, G.W. *A Handbook of Surgical Diathermy.* 1966. John Wright & Sons, Bristol, England.

Moritz, A.R. and Henriques, F.C. The relative importance of time and surface temperature in the causation of skin burns. *Am. J. Pathol.* 1947, 23: 605–720.

Overmeyer, K., Pearce, J.A., and DeWitt, D.P. Measurements of temperature distribution at electrosurgical dispersive electrode sites. *Trans. ASME* 1979, 101: 66–72.

Parker, E. O. Esophageal burn at the site of an esophageal temperature probe. *Anesthesiology* 1984, 61(1): 93–95.

Pearce, J.A. *Electrosurgery.* 1986. Chapman and Hall, London, 258.

Pearce, J.A., Geddes, L.A., Smith, J., et al. The performance of dry and gelled electrosurgical electrodes. *Proc. 31st ACEMB,* paper 25.2. 1978. Atlanta.

Pearce, J.A. and Geddes, L.A. The characteristics of capacitive electrosurgical dispersive electrodes. *Proc. 15th AAMI Conf.,* 1980, 15: 162.

Pearce, J.A., Geddes, L.A., Bourland, J.D., and Silva, L.F. The thermal behavior of electrolyte-coated metal-foil electrodes. *Med. Instrum.* 1979, 3(5): 298–300.

Pearce, J.A., Geddes, L.A., VanVleet, J., et al. Skin burns from electrosurgical electrodes. *Med. Instrum.* 1983, 17: 225–231.

Peterson, H.B., Ory, H.W., Greenspan, J.R., et al. Deaths associated with laparoscopic sterilization by unipolar electrocoagulation devices. *Am. J. Obst. Gyn.* 1981, January: 141–143.

Prentiss, G.W.H., Bethard, W.F., Boatwright, D.E., and Pennington, R.D. Massive adductor muscle contraction in transurethral surgery. *J. Urol.* 1965, 93: 263–271.

Ross, J.V. Explosion during electrocauterization of a rectal polyp. *Dis. Colon Rectum* 1961, 6: 364–366.

Schellhammer, P.F. Electrosurgery. *Urology* 1974, 3(3): 261–268.

Schwimmer, W.B. Electrosurgical burn injuries during laparoscopy sterilization. *Obst. Gynecol.* 1974, 24(4): 526.

Stewart, K.S., Pearson, J.F., Docker, M.F., et al. A possible hazard of laparoscopic sterilization. *Am. J. Obst. Gynecol.* 1973, 115(8): 1154–1157.

Strimling, B.S. Partial amputation of glans penis during Mogen clamp circumcision. *Pediatrics* 1996, 87(8)Part 1: 906–907.

Thomas, S.D. Eye injury during transurethral surgery. *J. Urol.* 1975, 114: 584–585.

Thompson, B.H. and Wheeless, C.P. Gastrointestinal complications of laparoscopy sterilization. *Obst. Gynecol.* 1973, 41: 669.

Tucker, R.D., Schmitt, O.H., Silvert, C.E., and Silvis, S.E. Demodulated low frequency currents from electrosurgical procedures. *Surg. Gynecol. Obst.* 1984, 159: 39–43.

Wald, A.S., Mazzia, V.D.B., and Spencer, F.C. Accidental burns. *J.A.M.A.* 1971, 217(7): 916–921.

Ward, G.E. An efficient method of hemostasis without suture. *Med. J. Record* 1925, 121: 470.

Woodward, N.W., Prevention of explosion while fulgurating polyps of the colon. *Dis. Colon and Rectum* 1961, 4: 32.

Zimmerman, K. Detonation of intestinal gas by an electrosurgical unit. *Southern Med. J.* 1959, 52: 605–608.

4 Anesthesia

CONTENTS

INTRODUCTION

At present in the U.S. there are about 20 million anesthetic procedures performed annually, and it is estimated that there are 5000 cases of brain damage associated with them. Most anesthesiologists believe that appropriate instrumental aids could reduce this number by about 85% and would allow better management of all anesthetic procedures. In fact, use of the pulse oximeter, which measures oxygen saturation, has dramatically improved assessment of the adequacy of respiratory function. The number of anesthetic mishaps that result in neurological deficit is unknown. During anesthesia, the anesthesiologist is the custodian of the patient's life and vigilance is the essential ingredient. As one experienced anesthesiologist put it, managing the depth of anesthesia is like flying an airplane; the pilot responds to all the cues that permit a smooth flight, but an unexpected storm can occur, and the pilot must rely on instrumental aids and good judgment to ensure a safe flight and smooth landing.

ANESTHESIA MACHINE

The anesthesia machine provides a metered amount of the anesthetic gases and oxygen, removes the expired carbon dioxide, and includes a low-resistance path to a collapsible reservoir to permit easy breathing of the gas mixture. Because most modern anesthetics are volatile liquids, a vaporizer is used to evaporate the liquid. The inspiratory reservoir is a collapsible bag that can be compressed manually to apply artificial respiration. Valves are included in the circuit to ensure unidirectional flow of the gas mixture. There are two types of anesthetic circuit (circle): (1) the vaporizer is in the circle and (2) the vaporizer is outside of the circle.

IN-CIRCUIT VAPORIZER ANESTHESIA MACHINE

Figure 1 illustrates the anesthetic circuit in which the vaporizer (Vap) is in the breathing circuit. Oxygen and sometimes another gas, such as nitrous oxide (N_2O), are delivered, being metered by flowmeters. Note that part of the inspired gas passes over the liquid anesthetic, which evaporates, and part of the inspired gas bypasses the liquid. The ratio of these two components determines the concentration of the anesthetic in the breathing circuit. Inspiratory (I) and expiratory (EX) check valves guarantee unidirectional gas flow. The carbon-dioxide absorber (CO_2A) removes the exhaled CO_2 from the breathing circuit. The absorber is soda lime with an indicator that changes color when the absorber is exhausted.

OUT-OF-CIRCUIT VAPORIZER ANESTHESIA MACHINE

Figure 2 illustrates the out-of-circuit vaporizer anesthesia machine, which has the same components except that the vaporized anesthetic is delivered into the breathing circuit by first passing oxygen (and sometimes N_2O) through the vaporizer (Vap). Again, the concentration of the anesthetic gas in the breathing circuit is determined by the proportion of gas that passes over the anesthetic liquid.

The breathing bag (B) serves several important functions. Because the system is closed, the flow of oxygen and other gases into the system must equal the amount absorbed by the subject plus the amount due to any leak. The inflow of gases is constant and occurs slowly. Inspiration requires a relatively large volume of gas in a short time; the breathing bag acts as a reservoir to accommodate the demand of inspiration. With excessive gas inflow, the pressure in the circuit will rise and the excess pressure valve (XP) will automatically open to reduce the pressure. For an

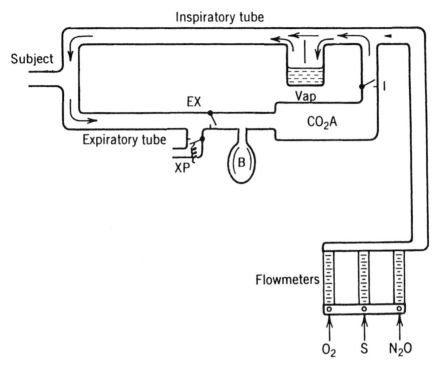

FIGURE 1   Anesthesia machine in which the vaporizer (Vap) is in the breathing circuit.

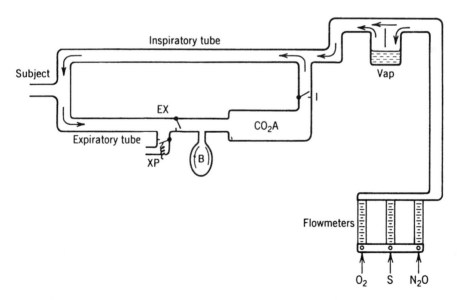

FIGURE 2   Anesthesia machine in which the vaporizer (Vap) is outside of the breathing circuit.

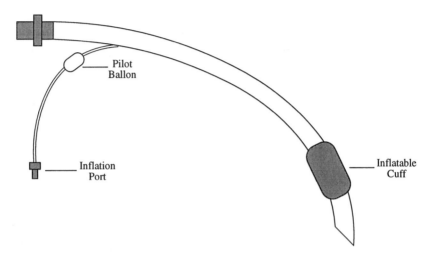

FIGURE 3 A typical disposable cuffed endotracheal tube with a pilot balloon to identify cuff inflation.

adult, the uptake of oxygen is about 300 ml/min, and the inflow is set at a value above that to accommodate metabolism and any leakage from the circuit.

The breathing bag also acts as an indicator of spontaneous respiration, decreasing in size during inspiration. Even more important, it affords a means for assisting respiration. Squeezing the bag forces gas into the lungs; releasing the bag allows the elastic recoil of the lungs and rib cage to effect expiration. The resistance offered to lung inflation informs the anesthetist about the airway compliance.

ENDOTRACHEAL TUBE

An endotracheal tube is placed in the trachea via the mouth to maintain an open airway. The tube may be cuffed or uncuffed; the inflatable cuff at the tip provides a leak-proof seal; Figure 3 illustrates a typical example. Such tubes are used with anesthesia machines and ventilators. Since the 1960s, sterilized, packaged, plastic disposable endotracheal tubes have been used. Prior to then, red rubber tubes were popular. There is an American Society for Testing Materials Standard (ASTM F1242-89) for endotracheal tubes.

Most modern disposable endotracheal tubes are of polyvinyl chloride (PVC); some are of silastic, which can be sterilized and reused. There are special endotracheal tubes for use with the laser, which produces a thermal pulse to cauterize tissue.

There are two scales for endotracheal tubes, the French (F) and the internal diameter in millimeters. The F scale identifies the outer diameter in millimeters and is this dimension multiplied by 3; i.e., a 10-mm-diameter endotracheal tube would be designated 30F.

As stated previously, the cuff at the tip of the endotracheal tube is inflated to provide a seal. Inflation with air (or sometimes saline) is via a port at the end of a tube in the wall of the endotracheal tube. A pilot balloon at the external (mouth) end of the tube allows identification that the cuff is inflated. The inflation pressure is an important factor because a pressure that is too high will impair the circulation of blood in the capillaries in the tracheal tissues embracing the cuff. Too low a pressure does not provide an adequate seal. A pressure of 25 to 35 cm H_2O is typical.

AUXILIARY EQUIPMENT

Associated with an anesthesia procedure are a variety of supporting devices, such as a ventilator and humidifier (which may or may not be a part of the anesthesia machine), a warming blanket, a warming cabinet to heat intravenous fluid containers, and a defibrillator for terminating cardiac arrhythmias. A typical ventilator consists of a flexible cylindrical bellows in a transparent chamber to which intermittent gas pressure is applied.

MONITORING EQUIPMENT

During anesthesia, both the anesthesia machine and the patient are monitored. Although the monitoring devices mounted on the anesthesia machine may sound an out-of-range alarm, those that are connected to the patient may or may not. Before describing the various monitoring systems, it is appropriate to recognize a recommendation by Satwicz and Shagrin (1981), who stated:

> The most useful monitoring is still done by sight, sound, smell, and touch, which requires physical proximity of the anesthesiologist to the patient.
>
> Ever-increasing amounts of electrical and mechanical devices are being marketed. These must be regarded as an extension of the anesthesiologist's discriminatory powers and not as a substitute for his decision-making processes. They must not detract from his direct observation of the patient.

ANESTHESIA -MACHINE MONITORING

Because anesthesia machines have a very long life, it is difficult to characterize the type of monitoring on a typical machine. Out-of-range alarms can be provided for the pressure in the breathing circuit, the concentration of oxygen and carbon dioxide in the circuit, oxygen/nitrous oxide ratio, and low oxygen pressure (after the regulator and before the flowmeters). Many of the monitoring devices are power-line operated and in case of a power failure, there is usually a backup battery supply. There is a trend to create pneumatically driven alarms. However, it is important to recognize that no electric power is needed to operate the basic anesthesia machines shown in Figures 1 and 2.

PATIENT MONITORING

The physiological events monitored during anesthesia depend, in part, on the nature and length of the procedure and the anesthesiologist's preference and experience. Typically the electrocardiogram (ECG) is monitored from chest electrodes. The ECG provides heart rate and can identify any abnormality in rhythm, as well as myocardial ischemia, revealed by a change of the S-T segment. Blood pressure is often obtained directly from an arterial line and often indirectly with a blood-pressure cuff. Systolic, mean, and diastolic pressure are obtained after the cuff has undergone an inflation and deflation cycle to seat the cuff. Central venous pressure (CVP) is often measured with a catheter advanced into a jugular vein. The oxygen saturation (redness of the blood) is measured noninvasively with a pulse oximeter applied to a fingertip. Some anesthesiologists place a tube in the esophagus and connect it to the stethoscope to monitor heart and breath sounds. Sometimes the stethoscope is taped to the upper chest over the trachea. Body temperature is also measured because anesthesia depresses the temperature-regulating capability of the body. Often an electronic thermometer is placed in the rectum or esophagus. If the procedure is long, blood gases (pH, pO_2, and pCO_2) will be determined from drawn blood samples, usually from the radial artery at the wrist. Airway carbon dioxide concentration is measured with an infrared analyzer; this technique is known as capnometry (capnos = smoke). The end-expiratory CO_2 reflects arterial pCO_2, which is a useful indicator of the metabolic state of the patient.

Some anesthesiologists monitor cardiac output noninvasively with the impedance cardiograph (see below), which employs passage of a low-intensity, high-frequency current through the chest by electrodes on the neck and thorax. Cardiac output is sometimes measured invasively with the thermodilution method, in which a bolus of chilled 5% dextrose in water (D5W) is injected into the right atrium and the transient decrease in blood temperature is measured in the pulmonary artery. Usually several injections are used to obtain a reliable value for assessing cardiac output.

ALARMS

By definition, an alarm is any sound, outcry, or information intended to give notice of approaching danger. Clearly, alarms are highly desirable during anesthesia. However, the most desirable alarm types (audible and/or visual) are the subject of considerable debate. Samuels (1986) pointed out that many of the audible alarms on different monitoring devices are similar, making it difficult to identify which physiological event or machine parameter is out of range.

There is an interesting background to alarms. For example, aviation cockpit alarms were standardized in civil aviation in the U.K. following the recommendation by Patterson (1982). According to Weinger (1991), these alarm tones were modified for the medical environment and consist of "well-defined, complex sequences of tones producing distinctive auditory signatures. There are three 'general' alarm sounds of increasing complexity for advisory, caution, and warning. Six 'specialized' alarm categories have been defined (ventilation, oxygenation, cardiovascular, perfusion, drug administration, and temperature), each with its own unique auditory signature. For each category, both a caution alarm and a warning alarm are specified."

In 1986 the American Society of Anesthesiologists published recommended standards for monitoring, which included arterial blood pressure, electrocardiography, an oxygen analyzer, and a ventilator disconnection alarm. Alarms are now included in pulse oximeters and are capnographs.

In 1993 the American Society for Testing Materials published alarm standards for anesthesia and respiratory care. The standard requires that alarm sounds have a fundamental frequency between 150 and 1000 Hz based on standard musical pitches. There must be at least four frequency components ranging from 300 to 4000 Hz and these must be related so that they form a distinct sound. Adjustable alarms must have an intensity between 45 and 85 dB. Those with fixed intensity must be between 70 and 85 dB.

Despite the fact that there are recommended standards for alarm signatures, not all anesthesia machines carry the same monitoring equipment; often what is installed reflects the preference and experience of the anesthesiologist. Moreover, all alarms are not equal; some represent a life-threatening emergency, while others may indicate a relatively benign condition. Therefore, prioritization and integration of alarms is an important consideration. The technology of alarming is evolving toward development of the "smart alarm" which, according to Dorsch and Dorsch (1994), "will identify the source of the alarm, analyze the data, provide the operator with a list of possible conditions that could have triggered the alarm, and may present information that will aid in determining the correct way to deal with the condition that triggered the alarm." Parenthetically, modern aircraft cockpit audible and visible alarms are converted to speech commands that are heard by the pilot in his/her headset. Feldman et al. (1985) advocated the use of synthetic speech as an alarm signal in anesthesia. Although there are recommendations for alarm standards, Weinger (1991) stated that the AAMI committee developing human factor guidelines for medical devices opposes rigidly defined alarm standards for medical equipment until more input is obtained from clinicians. Note that in the case of anesthesia alarms, three fields of instrumentation are involved: cardiovascular, respiratory, and anesthesia. In the meantime, the alarms on these three types of equipment sound separately.

The kinds of events that sound alarms were reviewed by McIntyre (1982), who surveyed members of the Canadian Anesthetists Society and reported that over half of the 852 respondents had deliberately deactivated audible alarms at the start of the anesthetic procedure and 314 (37%) stated that they did so because there were too many false alarms. Fifty-three respondents (6%) believed that the confusion between different audible signals made the alarm useless, while 45 (5%) believed that an audible alarm hindered patient care. In a study by Kestin et al. (1988) involving 50 patients undergoing pediatric anesthesia, a mean of ten alarms sounded during each procedure and 75% of these were spurious; only 3% indicated risk to the patient. Of all alarms, 99% were from the pulse oximeter, electrocardiogram, or blood-pressure monitors, although the alarm limits were set at values that most anesthetists would consider entirely appropriate for patients in this age group.

Another survey of alarm incidence was presented by Schaaf and Black (1989), who reported:

> The number of alarms averaged three per case, with a mean frequency of one every 34 minutes. Spurious alarms (those caused by electrocautery, accidental patient movement, or other nonphysiologic reasons) represented only 24% of all alarms. Those alarms sounding that were outside the limits occurred at a rate of 53% and

those that were considered patient risks occurred at a rate of 22%. Of the alarms, 67% occurred at the beginning and end of anesthesia. The end-tidal carbon dioxide reading accounted for 42% of the alarms, mostly during intubation and extubation. The other alarm percentages were as follows: inspired oxygen fraction, 2%; ECG heart rate, 5%; noninvasive blood pressure, 30%; and pulse oximeter, 20%.

As sources of artifact, Kestin et al. (1988) reported interference from the electro-cautery or operating room lights; both of these were causes of spurious alarms.

The status of alarms on the three types of monitoring equipment remains unsettled. It is hoped that the evolutionary path does not result in alarms that harm. For example, there is a loud cockpit horn that sounds when the throttle and wing flaps have a certain setting for landing and the landing gear is not extended. On one occasion the airport tower radio was calling the pilot to tell him that his landing gear was not down. The pilot could not hear the tower because the alarm horn was so loud.

While an ideal alarm system is being developed, it should be recognized that if artifacts cause alarms to sound repeatedly when there is no danger to the patient, the alarm is usually turned off. While this practice is common, the alarm may not be turned on again, which could be hazardous.

ANESTHESIA MACHINE MISHAPS

Despite the fact that monitoring equipment and alarms have been added to the anesthetic procedure, mishaps still occur. Arens (1996) analyzed the American Society of Anesthesiologists' (ASA) closed-claim files and reported "that 79% of claims related to equipment were due to misuse and 19% were due to equipment failure. In addition, modern anesthesia machines powered by electricity can immediately become a major problem in times of weather disasters and power outages, when backup generators may fail."

Arens went on to argue that overreliance on monitoring equipment leads to a reduction in vigilance and stated that "the anesthesiologist is the patient's most important monitor" and that the anesthesiologist should be in close contact with the patient at all times.

CARBON-DIOXIDE ABSORBER FAILURE

Exhaled carbon dioxide (CO_2) is absorbed chemically by soda lime that contains an indicator (e.g., ethyl violet) which turns purple when the absorber is exhausted. Carbon dioxide is a potent respiratory stimulus, causing the breathing rate and depth to increase. An increase in the concentration of CO_2 in the blood is known as hypercarbia. If this occurs when a spontaneously breathing patient is connected to an anesthesia machine, several undesirable consequences could occur, not the least of which is the inhalation of more anesthetic, thereby deepening the level of anesthesia.

Detmer et al. (1980) reported a case of hypercarbia due to carbon-dioxide absorber failure because of absence of the color indicator (ethyl violet) which signals exhaustion of the absorber. The hypercarbia was discovered by blood-gas analysis.

The event was not due to an oversight on the part of the manufacturer of the soda lime; the hospital had purchased industrial-grade soda lime, which has no color indicator.

Andrews et al. (1990) reported a case of CO_2 absorber failure due to deactivation of the color indicator by radiation from room fluorescent lights (which emit a small amount of ultraviolet radiation). They carried out a series of carefully controlled experiments and stated:

> After 24 h of fluorescent light exposure with a received flux density of 46 mwatts/cm^2 at 254 nm, the concentration of functional ethyl violet remaining in pulverized Sodasorb® was 16% of the baseline value. Furthermore, using multiple light sources of various intensities, the greater the intensity of light, the more rapid the rate of decline of the ethyl violet concentration.

Finally, they pointed out that:

> Photodeactivation is more likely to occur in operating rooms (OR) that are brightly lighted or in those that utilize UV germicidal bulbs. Intensely lighted OR is the trend, and many existing OR contain germicidal UV bulbs. End-tidal CO_2 monitoring may be more beneficial than color change of absorbent to diagnose rebreathing in those operating rooms.

VALVE MALFUNCTION

The function of the check valves is to guarantee unidirectional gas flow in the breathing circuit. If the valves do not close properly, rebreathing of CO_2 will result. Expiratory-valve failure was reported by Nunn and Rosewarne (1990), who observed an increase in airway CO_2 identified by the capnometer. The importance of incompetent valves was reported by Podraza et al. (1991), who examined the effect of removing the inspiratory and expiratory valves. Removal of the expiratory valve resulted in the greatest rebreathing of CO_2.

Hypercarbia can be detected by blood-gas analysis (pCO_2) and by capnometry. With continuous rebreathing, the end-tidal CO_2 will increase, alerting the anesthesiologists to the problem. Sticking valves were described by Parry et al. (1991) as a source of CO_2 buildup.

LEAKS AND DISCONNECTIONS

Leaks can occur anywhere in the breathing circuit and in the oxygen line. Leaks can be identified with the application of soapy water to the suspected leak site.

Although disconnections can occur anywhere in the breathing circuit, the most common site is between the endotracheal tube and the anesthesia machine. Typically, the tubing in the anesthetic circuit is held together by friction at the joints which may be plastic-to-plastic or metal-to-plastic. Some clamping devices as well as adhesive tape are used to secure these joints, the latter not being recommended because it makes reconnection more difficult. In many cases it is desirable to have an easy way of disconnecting the anesthesia machine from the tracheal tube to permit suction of mucous.

Accidental disconnection of the anesthesia machine at the tracheal tube is a serious mishap. Either of two events can occur: if the patient is breathing spontaneously, he/she will breathe room air and blow off the anesthesia gas, resulting in a lessening depth of anesthesia. If the patient was treated with a muscle relaxant, as occurs frequently, the respiratory muscles may be paralyzed and breathing can cease. The use of a muscle relaxant during anesthesia is quite common.

PULSE OXIMETER

INTRODUCTION

The pulse oximeter is an optical instrument that measures the redness of the blood, which depends on arterial oxygen saturation (S_aO_2), the measurement being made by a fiberoptic bundle. Because there is no electrical contact with the patient, there is minimal opportunity for an electrical hazard. However, small optical signals are involved and environmental interference can affect the accuracy of the saturation reading.

PRINCIPLE OF OPERATION

The pulse oximeter determines the oxygen saturation by measuring the optical transmission at two wavelengths (650 and 805 nm) of light passing through a tissue bed, usually the fingertip. Figure 4 illustrates the method by which one fiberoptic bundle transmits broadband radiation from a halogen lamp through the fingertip. A second fiberoptic bundle carries the transmitted light back to two optical filters which allow measurement of the transmission at 650 and 805 nm. The unique feature of the pulse oximeter is that the optical transmission measurement is made during each pulse and special electronic circuitry is used to make this beat-by-beat measurement, which is averaged. The oxygen saturation ($S_a O_2$) is proportional to the ratio of the optical density (Y) at 650 and 805 nm. The readout is in percent oxygen saturation. Most pulse oximeters also indicate heart rate and some display the pulse graphically.

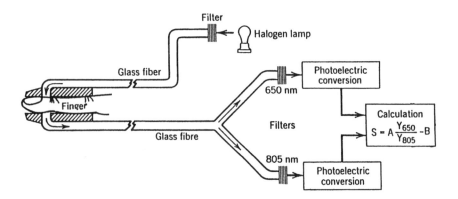

FIGURE 4   Components of the pulse oximeter. (Redrawn from Yoshiya, I. et al. *Med. Biol. Eng. Comput.* 1988, 18: 27–31.)

OXYGEN SATURATION

Oxygen saturation is defined as the ratio of oxygenated hemoglobin (HbO_2) to the total hemoglobin ($Hb + HbO_2$). The former is measured at 650 nm and the latter at 805 nm. In a normal subject the hemoglobin concentration is 15 g/100 ml blood. One gram of hemoglobin combines with 1.34 ml of oxygen; therefore, the oxygen content for 100% saturation is $15 \times 1.34 = 20.1$ ml O_2/100 ml blood. There is, in addition, a small amount of oxygen dissolved in the plasma. Note that if the hemoglobin concentration is less than normal, 100% saturation represents less than 20.1 ml O_2/100 ml blood.

OXYGEN DISSOCIATION CURVE

Oxygen saturation depends on the partial pressure of oxygen to which the blood is exposed. The concept of partial pressure is readily understood by the following example. If the barometric pressure is 760 mmHg, then 100% oxygen would have a partial pressure of 760 mmHg. If the gas sample has 20% oxygen, the partial pressure for a barometric pressure of 760 mmHg is 20% of 760 = 152 mmHg.

Figure 5 illustrates how the oxygen saturation increases with the partial pressure of oxygen (pO_2). The different curves are for blood pH of 7.2, 7.4, and 7.6. Note that with a normal pH = 7.40, 95% saturation is achieved with a $pO_2 = 80$ mmHg, i.e., $100 \times 80/760 = 10.5\%$ oxygen. Twenty percent oxygen ($pO_2 = 152$) provides an oxygen saturation of about 98% for a normal subject at 760 mmHg barometric pressure.

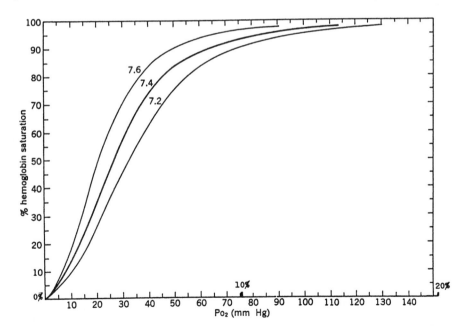

FIGURE 5 The relationship between oxygen saturation and partial pressure of oxygen and percent oxygen for different pH values (7.2, 7.4, 7.6).

HAZARDS AND ACCIDENTS WITH PULSE OXIMETRY

It would appear that there are few hazards associated with pulse oximetry; however, there have been a few disastrous fires, not due to the pulse oximeter, but associated with its use during anesthesia in the operating room. For example, a high concentration of oxygen (more than 80%) is typically used with anesthetic gases, and the oxygen flow for an adult is often 1 l/minute or more. This high flow and partial pressure guarantee high oxygen saturation, as predicted by Figure 5. Anesthesiologists like to keep the S_aO_2 as high as possible and use high oxygen flow to the anesthetic circuit. However, this practice is not without a fire hazard. An adult human consumes about one quarter liter of oxygen per minute. The oxygen flow rate into an anesthetic machine is often four to ten times this amount and the excess may leak into the environment if an open system is used and if the exhaled gases are not scavenged. The drapes over the patient can constitute an oxygen-filled tent. Despite the fact that drapes are treated with a flame retardant, there have been instances of the drapes catching fire when a small spark occurred. In one case, investigated by the author, under a poorly applied defibrillating electrode, a spark to the patient's skin caused the drapes to catch fire. Another instance of a fire was due to the leakage of oxygen around a plastic facemask and an electrosurgical spark ignited the drapes, and burned the patient, the facemask, and the surgeon's fingers.

An unusual type of incident occurred with a normally functioning pulse oximeter. Block and Stahl (1995) were monitoring oxygen saturation in an anesthetized patient. The control values were 96% saturation and 80 heartbeats/min. The efficacy of a muscle relaxant was assessed by applying electrical stimuli at 1/sec to a pair of electrodes placed across the elbow to cause the fingers of the hand to twitch. Immediately the pulse oximeter showed a saturation of 73%. The stimulator was turned off and the saturation returned to 98%. In explaining this incorrect indication of saturation, the authors stated:

> The technology of pulse oximetry depends upon the assumption that blood is the only substance that pulsates between the emitter and the detector of the oximeter. In the case presented here, the muscular contractions evoked by the nerve stimulator simulated a "pulse" at a frequency of 60 "beats"/min. These contractions caused obvious motion of the finger, which probably resulted in blood volume shifts larger than those caused by the small pulsations of the heartbeat in the finger. Alternatively, the contractions may have produced small motions or slippages between the oximeter probe and the finger.

In the foregoing case, had the authors not been so vigilant they might have increased the oxygen flow in an attempt to raise the saturation from its incorrectly indicated value of 73%. The result would have been more oxygen in the environment of the patient with an increase in the risk of fire or explosion. The obvious solution to this problem is to place the oximeter on a finger on the opposite hand.

Artifacts and alarm sounding can occur with pulse oximeters. For example, if the finger probe is on the same arm as is used to measure blood pressure with a cuff, the pulse signal will disappear during cuff inflation and deflation. Motion artifacts sometimes occur due to shivering during light anesthesia. A poorly applied probe is also a source of artifact. The use of electrosurgery nearby also disrupts normal operation of the pulse oximeter. Any or all of the foregoing may signal an alarm, which may or may not represent a threat to the patient.

IMPEDANCE CARDIOGRAPHY

Stroke volume and cardiac output are measured noninvasively by injecting a low-intensity, high-frequency current via neck and abdomen electrodes. Two sensing electrodes, placed between the current-injecting electrodes, detect a cardiac-induced, pulsatile impedance change that can be processed to obtain stroke volume and cardiac output when blood resistivity is known. Without knowing blood resistivity, impedance cardiography is useful for tracking changes in cardiac output.

Using impedance cardiography to monitor a patient with an implanted pacemaker during surgery, Aldrete et al. (1995) reported that the patient's heart rate increased to 120/min. Drug therapy failed to reduce it and the ECG showed pacemaker spikes at 120/min. When the impedance cardiograph was disconnected, the heart rate returned to 72/min. The event occurred a second time.

Worthy of note is the fact that the 2.5-mA, 70-kHz current applied for impedance cardiography gained access to the pacemaker via the pacing electrodes, which are virtually in line with the 70-kHz current path. The pacemaker was of the programmable type and had been operating properly for 11 months prior to the event. It is clear that the 70-kHz current caused the pacemaker rate to increase from 72 to 120 beats/min. Neither the instruction manual for the pacemaker, nor that for the impedance cardiograph identified this hazard.

BURNS FROM WARMING DEVICES

During general anesthesia, the body's temperature-regulating mechanism is depressed and body temperature decreases. Contributing to this decline is the relatively cool environment of the operating room. Therefore, a variety of devices, such as warmed mattresses, hot-water bottles and bags, heat lamps, heated humidifiers, forced-air warming blankets, etc. are employed. Burns have been associated with the use of some of these warming devices.

Cheney et al. (1994) reviewed the Closed Claims Database of the American Society of Anesthesiologists which lists a total of 3000 claims (1985–1994) of which 54 were burn cases, and of these, 28 resulted from materials or devices used to warm patients; Table 1 presents their results. Cheney et al. stated:

> Among the 18 burns caused by a heated i.v. bag or bottle, 15 involved an i.v. bag or bottle being used to warm the patient (14 directly and 1 by warming an i.v. blood transfusion). In the other three claims, a warmed i.v. bag or bottle was placed on the patient's skin in order to provide local heat. In 5 of the 18 burns caused by i.v. bags or bottles, the reviewer explicitly stated that the burn was of second or third-degree severity.

TABLE 1
Source of Burns from Warming Devices

	N	% of 28
Heated material	20	71
i.v. bag/bottle	18	64
Hot packs/compresses	2	7
Warming equipment	8	29
Circulating water blanket	5	18
Warming light	1	4
Heated humidifier	1	4
Heating pad	1	4

From Cheney, F.W., Posner, K.L., Caplan, R.A., et al.
Anesthesiology 1994, 80: 806–810.

Burns from electrically powered warming equipment represent only 29% of the total burns from warming devices. More than half of the burns in this category were from circulating-water mattresses. In only one of the burns caused by circulating-water mattresses did the reviewer explicitly state that the device was defective.

Of more than passing interest are the circumstances surrounding the incidents. According to Cheney et al. (1994):

One burn resulted from a warming light that was being used to treat hypothermia in a 2-day-old infant. The anesthesiologist had removed the diffusing lens from the lamp and placed the lamp 3 m from the patient. The infant sustained third-degree burns despite constant vigilance over skin temperature.

One burn was caused by a heated humidifier. The tubing was padded but came in contact with the arm and a permanent disfiguring scar resulted. The one heating pad burn resulted from treatment of an i.v. infiltration. The patient sustained scars and underwent multiple surgical procedures.

The data base contained five burns from heated i.v. fluid bags used to posture patients during surgery. The following case provides an example of such an incident.

Pamaar et al. (1992) reported a second-degree burn on the back of the neck when a heated bag of intravenous fluid (IVF) was used to hyperextend the neck. They stated:

A thirty-year-old, 70-kg woman, ASA physical status 1, was admitted for elective tonsillectomy. Under general anesthesia, the patient was positioned supine with both arms tucked by her sides. The neck was hyperextended by placing a 1-l bag of IVF between the scapulae. The IVF bag was placed on top of a heating blanket warmed to 39°C. Two layers of cotton sheets were between the patient and the IVF bag. Surgery proceeded for 30 min, and after uneventful extubation and emergence, the patient was brought to the recovery room. Fifteen minutes later the patient complained of pain and burning sensations across the upper back. Examination at this time revealed a 10 × 30-cm area of second-degree burn with blistering, transversely across the upper back. The outline of the injury corresponded to the position and shape of the IVF bag.

Not content to accept the physical evidence alone, Pamaar et al. further investigated the accident and stated:

> We attempted to simulate the events surrounding the injury. A heated IVF bag from the same warmer was used to support the shoulders of an awake volunteer. Although only warm to the touch, the IVF bag was uncomfortably hot when laid upon, and the pain was intolerable after 10 min. The temperature of this IVF bag was 48°C at the outset and decreased only 3.2°C during 30 min. of exposure to the warming blanket. The blanket apparently limited the dissipation of heat from the IVF. Both pressure and persistent heat likely contributed to the burn in our patient.

FIRE

INTRODUCTION

For a fire to occur, three ingredients must be present: (1) a source of flammable material, (2) oxygen, and (3) a source of ignition (i.e., a spark or high temperature as produced by a laser beam). In the operating room all three ingredients can be present and circumstances can conspire to cause a fire or explosion.

Typically during anesthesia, 80 to 95% oxygen is used with the anesthetic agent applied to the airway via a plastic endotracheal tube. Occasionally, there may be a leak in the anesthetic circuit and thus oxygen may accumulate around the patient, who is covered with sterile paper or cloth drapes which are usually treated with a flame retardant. As stated previously, it is not uncommon for the flow of oxygen to be 1 l/min or more. An adult subject consumes about 0.25 to 0.3 l/min; therefore, the excess oxygen can accumulate in the environment providing the opportunity for a fire. The following cases are examples of fires in which all three ingredients were present.

DEFIBRILLATOR -INDUCED FIRE

The author investigated a case in which a defibrillation shock was delivered to two chest electrodes, one of which was not well applied and there was an arc under this electrode; the result was a flash that ignited the drapes, even though they were treated with a flame retardant. There is no arc under properly applied defibrillating electrodes.

ENDOTRACHEAL TUBE FIRE

A case investigated by the author involved an anesthetized subject with a plastic tracheal tube in place and the surgeon entered the trachea with an electrosurgical probe via a tracheostomy. The combination of a spark, oxygen, and an flammable material (plastic tracheal tube) resulted in an explosion, melting the anesthetic-machine tubes and burning the patient.

The use of a urethral resectoscope to eliminate obstructions in the airway was introduced by Johnson and Stewart (1975). Resection is achieved with electrosurgical current and when used in urological practice, only tissue and fluid surround the cutting loop. When used in the airway, tissue and oxygen surround the cutting loop.

Downing and Johnson (1979) reported successful use of an infant urethral resectoscope to excise subglottic stenoses in 22 infants. They described the resectoscope as follows:

> The instrument we use is an infant urethral resectoscope with a size 13 insulated sheath (3.5 × 4.2 mm O.D.) and a 0° rod lens telescope with fiberoptic illumination. Ventilation can be achieved for a limited period of time when working without a tracheostomy by using a semi-closed system attached to the irrigating channel of the resectoscope sheath. Under such conditions, the endoscopic manipulations must be performed rapidly and at several short intervals. We have used intra-operative blood-gas monitoring with computer automated rapid analysis when working under these conditions without a tracheostomy.

Commenting on the results, Downing and Johnson stated:

> Twenty patients have had a successful clinical result with no evidence of recurrent airway stenosis. The result was unsuccessful in two patients, 1 of whom re-stenosed and has subsequently been retreated and decannulated successfully. The second patient re-stenosed and still has a tracheostomy. There were no deaths directly related to the resection procedure.

It is of more than passing interest to note that Downing and Johnson did not encounter a fire or explosion, which was reported by subsequent clinicians using the same technique (see below). The lack of fire or explosion may have been due to the absence of combustible material in the operating field. Although they reported using a suction cannula, they did not identify its construction. Because no fire was encountered, it is likely that the cannula was made of metal. As discovered by subsequent clinicians, the combination of oxygen, a plastic catheter, and an electrosurgical spark constitutes the ingredients for a fire.

Rita and Seleny (1982) reported an electrosurgically-induced endotracheal tube fire when they used a urethral resectoscope to remove granulous tissue in the trachea of a 12-year-old child. They reported:

> Bronchoscopy and tracheal dilatations had been done periodically under general anesthesia. The same technique has always been employed without complications, namely, passing an endotracheal tube through the tracheostomy. Anesthesia was induced and maintained by inhalation of halothane and 50% nitrous oxide. The last four procedures included removal of granulation tissue found at the tracheostomy site which was resected with the urethral resectoscope. No complications had occurred.
>
> This time, the same procedure was followed. Atropine, 0.2 mg, was administered intramuscularly 1 h before inducing anesthesia with halothane and 50 percent nitrous oxide through the tracheostomy tube. When adequate anesthetic depth was attained, the epiglottis, arytenoids, vocal cords, and trachea were sprayed with 1 percent

lidocaine. The tracheostomy tube was removed and a plastic endotracheal tube was passed through the tracheostomy. During bronchoscopy, granulation tissue was found at the tracheostomy site in the area above the endotracheal tube. While resecting it with the urethral resectoscope, smoke suddenly came out of the child's mouth and we saw a flash at the tracheostomy site. The endotracheal tube was immediately withdrawn. It was on fire which rapidly ceased spontaneously. Bronchoscopy showed burns on the lower trachea and right bronchus, with minimal involvement of the left bronchus.

Interestingly, they commented as follows:

In the past year, we have done 67 cases under general anesthesia without complications using halothane, 50 percent nitrous oxide, and an endotracheal tube inserted through the tracheostomy. This time, ignition of an endotracheal tube occurred during resection of tracheal granuloma using a urethral resectoscope.

From the foregoing case it is clear that the three ingredients for a fire were present: (1) a combustible substance, (2) oxygen, and (3) a source of ignition. It is surprising that these three ingredients were present 67 times during the last year and no fire occurred, indicating that if the three ingredients are present, sooner or later a fire will occur.

Another electrosurgically-induced tracheal tube fire was reported by Simpson and Wolf (1986), who stated:

A 4-yr-old boy was admitted for elective adenoidectomy and tonsillectomy. His past medical history was negative except for recurrent tonsillitis, the last episode having occurred 3 to 4 weeks prior to surgery... He weighed 17 kg and his physical examination was normal except for large, opposed tonsils touching at the midline.

Anesthesia was induced by inhalation of O_2, N_2O, and halothane and was uneventful. An i.v. infusion was then started. The trachea was automatically intubated with a 4.5 mm ID polyvinyl chloride (PVC) endotracheal tube. Lubricant was not used on the endotracheal tube. Breath sounds were equal bilaterally in all four quadrants. The endotracheal tube was fixed with the aid of a David-Crow mouth gag. Endotracheal tube position was again confirmed by equal breath sounds bilaterally. The eyes were protected with tape. The patient breathed N_2O 3L/min, O_2 3L/min, and 1% halothane, by controlled ventilation. A moderate retrograde leak of gases was noted around the tube at the larynx.

The surgeons performed the adenoidectomy and right tonsillectomy without incident, then began to use a suction and electrocautery to control the bleeding in the right tonsillar fossa. The electrocautery was set at 35-watts coagulation in the "spray" mode. After approximately 20 sec of cautery, a fire erupted in the pharynx that "blow-torched" toward the lips. Breath sounds were immediately lost and increased airway pressure was noted. The fire was extinguished with saline, the pharynx was suctioned, and the endotracheal tube was immediately removed. The tube was noted to be melted and charred externally for 2 cm, midway between the distal tip and the adaptor, and fused for 1 cm at that point with 100% occlusion. From the point of fusion distally, the tube was blackened internally. The trachea was immediately reintubated with a 5.0 mm ID PVC, uncuffed, endotracheal tube. With a fractional inspired O_2 concentration (F_1O_2) of 0.99 and 1% halothane, pH was 7.43,

Pa_{CO_2} 28 mmHg, and Pa_{O_2} 575 mmHg. On direct examination the mucosa of the posterior tongue, uvula, and hypopharynx was noted to be erythematous and charred. Rigid bronchoscopy using a 4.0 mm × 30 cm bronchoscope was performed. The cords were not burned, but were edematous. The mucosa of the anterior trachea, carina, and left mainstem bronchus was erythematous and charred in some areas. This was probably caused by a "blow-torching" of the fire downward. The burns were mostly anterior and not circumferential. After bronchoscopy, the trachea was reintubated orally with a 5.0 mm ID PVC, uncuffed, endotracheal tube under direct vision. Breath sounds were again equal and clear bilaterally. The patient was given dexamethasone 2 mg iv. Ours is the first reported case of an endotracheal tube fire ignited by "spray-type" coagulation cautery.

LASER-INDUCED FIRE

After performing 700 endotracheal and laryngeal procedures over a 3-year period, Snow et al. (1976) reported two cases of laser-induced tracheal tube fire using a red-rubber endotracheal tube. The first case was a 12-month-old girl. They reported:

> The larynx was exposed with a pediatric laryngoscope and placed on the suspension apparatus. A Zeiss operating microscope with laser attachment was brought into position.
>
> When the laser beam was continuously discharged, the papillomas obstructing the larynx were vaporized, so that the laser beam impacted on the tube within the trachea at the tracheotomy level. A fire started, which was brought under control immediately, by removal of the burning tube. Examination of the endotracheal tube revealed a superficial burned area, 1 × 0.5 cm in size, 4 cm from the distal end. Bronchoscopy revealed a small superficial burn of the tracheal mucosa, which later healed.

The second case was a 12-year-old boy with laryngial papillomas. The red-rubber endotracheal tube was covered with aluminum foil, except for the tip. They stated:

> During the operation, laser beam repeatedly hit the unprotected distal end of the tube. A fire started, which was brought under control immediately by removal of the burning tube. Examination of the tube showed a superficial burned area, 1.2 × 0.5 cm in size, including the aperture opposite the beveled end of the endotracheal tube. Bronchoscopy revealed a small superficial burn of the tracheal mucosa, 1 cm below the vocal cords, which healed uneventfully.

In commenting on their experience, they stated:

> During CO_2 laser microsurgery on the larynx and trachea, we have observed that if the laser beam repeatedly hits the red-rubber Rusch endotracheal tube (four or five times) in the same area, there is the risk of fire. The laser beam must be carefully focused to avoid impact with the tube.

Despite the aluminum foil used to protect the rubber tracheal tube, the unprotected tip was struck and the combustible rubber, in the presence of oxygen, caused a fire.

By 1979, it was recognized that a plastic tracheal tube in the airway could be ignited by a laser beam. Desirous of preventing such an event, Burgess and LeJune (1979) wrapped a polyvinyl tracheal tube with aluminum foil tape to within 1 cm of its tip. Despite this precaution, a laser-induced endotracheal tube fire occurred in a 6-year-old girl admitted for resection of papillomas on the left and right vocal cords. After induction of anesthesia and placement of the tracheal tube, Burgess and LeJune stated:

> When the papillomas that extended into the subglottic region were excised, however, heat from the laser beam melted and then ignited the endotracheal tube tip, which had become exposed below the area that was protected by tape. The tube was immediately withdrawn.
>
> Careful inspection of the trachea with a 5-mm bronchoscope showed no significant thermal injury in the subglottic area. Indeed, the area appeared to be notably improved by the surgery. The patient's trachea was reintubated, and the oropharynx was inspected and found to be uninjured. To prevent inflammation, dexamethasone, 8 mg i.v., was given intraoperatively and continued for two days postoperatively in a dose of 2 mg i.v. every 6 h. The three loose teeth were carefully extracted to prevent their being aspirated into the tracheobronchial tree. The trachea was extubated and the patient was given cool mist oxygen (40%) for the next 48 h. Arterial blood gases remained satisfactory. Ampicillin sodium, 250 mg four times daily, was administered for the next ten days. The patient's voice continued to improve over the next three weeks.

Another laser-induced endotracheal tube fire was reported by Hirshman and Smith (1980). The patient was a 14-year-old-boy with a tracheostomy who had 110 previous operations for tracheal and laryngeal papillomas (finger-like tumors). After sedation, they stated:

> The trachea was intubated via the larynx with a 6-mm-cuffed vinyl plastic endotracheal tube that was positioned just below the vocal cords to allow laser removal of the tracheal papillomas via the tracheal stoma. After spontaneous ventilation returned, the patient was allowed to breathe oxygen (O_2), nitrous oxide (N_2O) (50:50), and 2% halothane. Using a nasal speculum in the tracheal stoma, the CO_2 laser was used in 0.2-s bursts to remove several papillomas in the tracheal stoma entrance. After the papillomas in the stoma were removed, several large pedunculated papillomas were removed with cup forceps, and the bases were treated with the CO_2 laser, set at 0.5 s. All papillomas were removed from the right lateral wall. This took approximately ten minutes and, during this time, it was noted that the carbon/eschar from previously lasered areas produced sparks. Attention was then focused on the left lateral wall. After half of the first papilloma was removed, a hissing and then a small explosion were heard. The hoses from the anesthesia machine were immediately disconnected, the endotracheal tube was removed, the tracheostomy site was intubated with another tube, and 100% O_2 was administered.
>
> Vital signs were stable. A bronchoscope was used to inspect the larynx, which was free of damage. The trachea, however, showed a burn of the anterior wall, approximately 0.5 cm wide, beginning below the vocal cords to just above the tracheostomy site. There was also a small burned area 2.5 cm long and 1.2 cm wide above the tracheostomy on the posterior wall.

With careful medical management, the patient was discharged from the hospital on the following day. In explaining the accident, Hirshman and Smith stated:

We are postulating that the vinyl plastic endotracheal tube was ignited by flaming tissue either in close proximity to or inhaled into the tip of the endotracheal tube during spontaneous ventilation with gases that support combustion.

In an editorial comment by Strong (1980), which followed the Hirshman and Smith paper, it states:

Fortunately, the problem can now be avoided by using a bronchoscope with a laser attachment or a stainless steel flexible endotracheal tube, both of which are now commercially available. These steel instruments are, of course, noncombustible in air or 100% oxygen (O_2) when impacted with laser energy currently in use in surgery.

The flexible, stainless-steel endotracheal tube referred to by Strong was described by Norton and DeVos (1978). The device was made from stripwound hose using stainless steel or, as an alternative, wire-wound square spring. The tube was wire brushed or matte finished to diminish light reflection into the surgeon's field of vision. Dorsch and Dorsch (1994) pointed out that many airway tubes designed for use with lasers are not entirely metal; some have plastic tips and cuffs. A laser strike on these parts, in the presence of oxygen, could ignite a fire. Moreover, such tubes are not as easy to manipulate and are not as smooth as conventional, all-plastic tubes.

A fire associated with the use of a laryngoscope was reported by Wegrzynowicz et al. (1992), who stated:

A 25-year-old man presented for laser ablation of recurrent laryngeal papillomata. History and physical examination were unremarkable other than a 20-pack/yr smoking history, a bushy mustache, and a weight of 129 kg. Anesthesia was induced with thiopental and Fentanyl. Ventilation via mask with oxygen, nitrous oxide, and isoflurane was without difficulty. Vecuronium was given to provide relaxation. The surgeon inserted an adult Dedo laryngoscope, and jet ventilation was instituted with oxygen via a 13-G cannula inserted in the left light-carrier channel of the Dedo laryngoscope. A thumb-controlled valve and 50-psi oxygen powered the jet (were used).

The patient's face and the perioral area were covered with soaking wet towels such that only the barrel of the Dedo laryngoscope was visible. Anesthesia was maintained with thiopental and Fentanyl during jet ventilation. There were no intraoperative problems except for brief periods of decreased hemoglobin oxygen saturation measured by pulse oximetry (S) during some episodes of apnea that were requested by the surgeon to eliminate movement of the vocal cords.

Near the end of the surgical procedure, the surgeon suddenly yelled "fire", and bright blue and orange flames accompanied by a muffled roar were observed coming up through and around the laryngoscope. Jet ventilation was stopped; the towels were removed and the patient's blazing mustache was extinguished with the wet towels. The surgeon, who was in a great deal of pain, noted that the latex glove had been burned away from two of the fingertips of his right hand. The Dedo laryngoscope was removed, and bag-and-mask ventilation was commenced. Subsequent rigid bronchoscopy revealed no carbonaceous material in the trachea, and except for evidence of lasering, the glottis was normal. Muscle relaxation was reversed and the patient was awakened. Recovery from anesthesia was otherwise unremarkable.

The patient suffered second-degree burns to his right upper lip and nasal rim. These were treated with 1% silver sulfadiazine (Silvadine) and healed over the next 2 weeks without further incident. The only other evidence of airway fire was burned nasal hair. The surgeon suffered second-degree burns to the right index and middle fingers that were severe enough to prevent him from operating for a week.

This patient experienced an unusual complication. An errant laser strike on the surgeon's latex glove ignited the glove, producing hot volatile fuel that was entrained by the jet ventilator. Combustion of the vaporized latex accelerated dramatically in the oxygen-enriched atmosphere of the airway. The gaseous products of combustion escaped through either the patient's nose or mouth and in turn ignited his mustache, despite the "protective" wet drapes. It would be impossible to determine to what degree the patient's mustache contributed to his facial burns, or whether combustion alone under the drapes would have been adequate to cause the degree of injury sustained.

CONCLUSION

As stated previously, a fire can occur when oxygen, a flammable material, and a source of ignition are present. Common sources of ignition are an electrostatic discharge, a spark from an electrosurgical electrode, and a pulse of laser energy. Sparking thermostat and motor starters used to be common ignition sources, but technology has changed and fewer such sources are encountered nowadays.

REFERENCES

AAMI — Association for the Advancement of Medical Instrumentation. 3330 Washington Boulevard, Arlington, VA 22201-4598.

Aldrete, A., Brown, C., Daily, J., et al. Pacemaker malfunction due to microcurrent injection from a bioimpedance noninvasive cardiac output monitor. *J. Clin. Mon.* 1995, 1(2): 131–133.

American Society of Anesthesiologists. *Newsletter,* 50: 12, 12, 1986. 520 N. Northwest Highway, Park Ridge, IL 60068-2573.

American Society for Testing and Materials. Standard specification for cuffed and uncuffed tracheal tubes (ASTM F1242-89) Philadelphia.

Andrews, J.J., Johnston, R.V., Bee, D.E., and Arens, J.F. Photodeactivation of ethyl violet. A potential hazard of sodasorb. *Anesthesiology* 1990, 72: 59–64.

Arens, J.F. Pro: there is nothing wrong with old anesthesia machines and equipment. *J. Clin. Mon.* 1996, 12: 37–38.

Block, F.E. and Stahl, D. Interference in a pulse oximeter from a nerve stimulator. *J. Clin Mon.* 1995, 11: 392–393.

Burgess, C.G. and LeJune, F.E. Endotracheal tube ignition during laser surgery of the larynx. *Arch. Otolaryngol.* 1979, 105: 561–562.

Cheney, F.W., Posner, K.L., Caplan, R.A., et al. Burns from warming devices in anesthesia. *Anesthesiology* 1994, 80: 806–810.

Detmer, M.D., Chandra, P., and Cohen, P.J. Occurrence of hypercarbia due to an unusual failure of anesthetic equipment. *Anesthesiology* 1980, 52: 278–279.

Dorsch, J.A. and Dorsch, S.E. *Understanding Anesthesia Equipment.* 3rd ed. 1994. Williams & Wilkins, Baltimore.

Downing, T.P. and Johnson, D.G. Excision of subglottic stenoses with the urethral resectoscope. *J. Pediatr. Surg.* 1979, 14(3): 252–257.

Feldman, J.M., Pugh, G., Gravenstein, J.S., et al. Automated data presentation using synthetic voice. *J. Clin.Mon.* 1985, 1: 283.

Hirshman, C.A. and Smith, J. Indirect ignition of the endotracheal tube during carbon dioxide laser surgery. *Arch. Otolaryngol.* 1980, 106: 639–641.

Johnson, D.G. and Stewart, D.R. Management of acquired tracheal obstructions in infancy. *J. Pediatr. Surg.* 1975, 10: 709–719.

Kestin, I.G., Miller, B.R., and Lockhart, C.H. Auditing alarms during anesthesia monitoring. *Anesthesiology* 1988, 69(1): 106–109.

McIntyre, J.W.R. Ergonomics: anesthetists' use of auditory alarms in the operating room. *J. Clin. Mon. Comput.* 1985, 2: 47–55.

Norton, M.L. and DeVos, P. Endotracheal tube for laser surgery of the larynx. *Ann. Otol.* 1978, 87: 554–557.

Nunn, B.J. and Rosewarne, F.A. Expiratory valve failure. *Anaesth. Intensive Care* 1990, 18: 273–274.

Pamaar, C.G., Ahmad, I., and Marsh, N.J. Accidental burn during tonsillectomy. *Anesthesiology* 1992, 76: 869.

Patterson, R.D. Guidelines for auditory warning systems in civil aircraft. Paper 82017 Aviation Authority. London, England. 1982.

Parry, T.M., Jewkes, D.A., and Smith, M. A sticking flutter valve. *Anaesthesia* (American Society of Anesthesiologists [ASA] 1991, 46: 229.

Podraza, A.G., Salem, M.R., Joseph, N.J., and Brenchley, J.L. Rebreathing due to incompetent unidirectional valves in the circle absorber system. *Anesthesiology* 1991, 75: A422.

Rita, L. and Seleny, F. Endotracheal tube ignition during laryngeal surgery with resectoscope. *Anesthesiology* 1982, 56: 60–61.

Samuels, S.J. Letter to the editor. *Anesthesiol.* 1986, 64: 128.

Schaaf, C. and Black, F.E. Evaluation of alarm sounds in the operating room. *J. Clin. Mon.* 1989, 5(4): 300–301.

Satwicz, P.R. and Shagrin, J.M. The selection of anesthetic equipment. *Int. Anesthesiol. Clin.* 1981, 19(2): 97–111.

Simpson, J. and Wolf, G.L. Endotracheal tube fire ignited by pharyngeal electrocautery. *Anesthesiology* 1986, 63: 76–77.

Snow, J.C., Norton, M.L., Tejinder, S.S., et al. Fire hazard during CO_2 laser microsurgery on the larynx and trachea. *Anesth. Analg.*1976, 55(1): 146–147.

Strong, M.S. Editorial comment. *Arch. Otolaryngol.* 1980, 106: 641.

Weinger, M.B. Proposed new alarm standards may make a bad situation worse. *Anesthesiology* 1991, 74: 791.

Wegrzynowicz, E., Jensen, N.F., Pearson, K., et al. Airway fire during jet ventrilation for laser excision of vocal cord papilloma. *Anesthesiology* 1992, 76: 468–469.

5 Catheter Accidents

CONTENTS

INTRODUCTION

Catheters have been used in medicine for therapy and diagnosis since Egyptian medicine in the time of the Pharaohs. Modern sterilized disposable catheters appeared in the 1950s. Catheter electrodes appeared with evolution of the cardiac pacemaker in the early 1960s. Catheters are placed in every body opening, as well as through surgically made openings. Blood vessels, ducts, and body cavities are all catheterized for sampling fluids, pressures, or to inject substances. Catheters are also used to remove materials such as stones. Electric current can gain access to internal body sites via the conductivity of the fluid in a catheter. Catheters can induce clots and emboli; they can fracture, break, and migrate, and examples of these events will be given in this chapter.

INTRAVASCULAR CATHETER INCIDENTS

CATHETER PINCHOFF

Accompanying the use of venous-access catheters for chronic delivery of medications are a variety of hazards such as blockage, breakage, embolization, and infection. Careful catheter management has minimized such events; however, a few still occur.

Fracture of a venous-access catheter was reported by Prager and Hintzberg (1987), who wrote:

> On May 23, 1984, a subcutaneous venous access device (Infusaport, Infusaid Corporation Norwood, MA) was implanted over the left anterior chest wall. No sutures were used to stabilize the catheter to the subclavian vein. The implantation site was

overlying the second left rib laterally and inferior to the lateral one-third of the left clavicle. Subsequently, the patient received multidrug chemotherapy and had a documented complete response to the drug treatment program. On March 7, 1985, 10 months after port placement, the patient experienced the sudden onset of bilateral chest pain. Physical examination revealed a patient in evident pain with an unremarkable subcutaneous disc access noted over the left anterior chest wall. Chest X-ray revealed an embolized catheter in the left pulmonary artery area. The catheter was removed the same day from the left pulmonary artery, using a percutaneous approach through the right subclavian vein. The embolized catheter fragment was retrieved under fluoroscopy guidance, using a No. 8.3 medium Stertzer (USCI Corporation, Billerica, MD) catheter with a 0.25 guide wire fashioned to form a snare.

Examination of the broken catheter segment revealed that the embolized portion of the catheter is not circular in cross-section, but instead has an elliptical configuration. Indeed, when one of the catheter pieces is rotated 90° relative to the mating half, the difference in cross-section shape is readily apparent.

Later, the type of compression fracture became known as "pinchoff" and it was attributed to compression of the catheter by the clavicle and first rib. Figure 1 shows the anatomic details of the clavicle, first rib, and associated veins. The region where pinchoff can be avoided is identified, along with the recommended catheter-entry region.

This author investigated a similar catheter accident that occurred to a 35-year-old lady who was receiving chronic intravenous drug therapy for cancer via a Groshong-valved catheter, the tip of which had been placed in the superior vena cava. The insertion was made via the left subclavian vein. A venogram showed that the catheter was patent. Some time later, the patient complained of chest pain, shortness of breath, rapid irregular heart rate, and she was diaphoretic when admitted to the emergency room. Her symptoms were strikingly similar to those of a heart attack. Radiological examination revealed a 4-in. segment of broken catheter in the right ventricle. The report stated:

> The patient was brought to the cardiac catheterization laboratory and prepped and draped in sterile fashion. Local anesthesia was obtained over the right femoral vein with 1% plain Lidocaine after which an 8 French hemostasis sheath was placed into the right femoral vein by modified Seldinger technique. Next, a four-prong grasping forcep was used to retrieve the catheter fragment under fluoroscopic guidance. The catheter fragment forcep and hemostasis sheath were all removed as one piece. Fluoroscopy demonstrated no residual catheter fragment. Complete hemostasis was achieved by direct pressure over the site for 10 minutes. The patient was returned to her room in stable condition.

The author had the opportunity to examine the explanted catheter fragment. The piece that broke off was 12.2 cm long and exhibited a pinched or flattened region where it broke. The tip having been originally placed in the superior vena cava, a breakage would cause blood flow to carry the broken segment into the right ventricle. With the continued beating of the heart, the broken segment acted as a mechanical stimulus and produced ectopic beats and runs of tachycardia, which reduced cardiac output leading to reduced coronary perfusion, hence the chest pain.

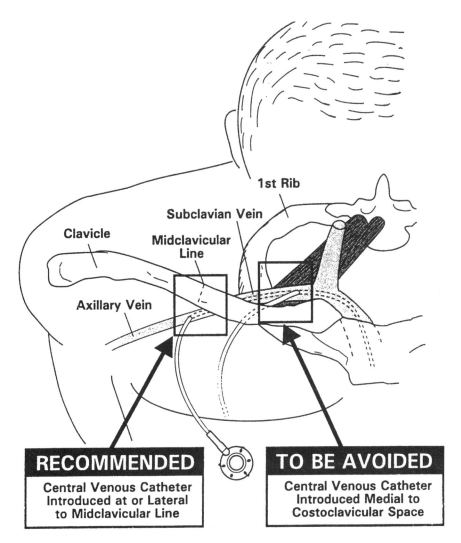

1st Rib

Subclavian Vein

Clavicle

Midclavicular Line

Axillary Vein

RECOMMENDED

Central Venous Catheter
Introduced at or Lateral
to Midclavicular Line

TO BE AVOIDED

Central Venous Catheter
Introduced Medial to
Costoclavicular Space

FIGURE 1 Anatomical details of the clavicle, first rib, and associated veins, identifying recommended catheter entry site and region to be avoided. (Courtesy of Cook Pacemaker Corp. Leechburg, PA 15656.)

The manufacturer's instructions carry a warning that identifies catheter pinchoff; it stated:

> When placing the catheter in the axillary-subclavian vein, insert the catheter into the vein at a point lateral to the angle between the clavicle and the first rib to avoid pinchoff of the catheter which may cause occlusion, damage, or breakage.

In the manufacturer's instructions, reference was made to a report by Aitken and Minton (1984), who studied 48 patients undergoing intravenous chemotherapy, and it stated:

4 of the patients had partial catheter obstruction owing to a pincher action of the clavicle and first rib. The roenterographic presence of the pinch-off sign indicates serious potential problems with the central venous Silastic catheter and is an indication for immediate catheter removal and replacement at another site or position. The other catheter entry sites recommended were a more lateral site or entry into the subclavian, cephalic, or internal jugular vein.

A catheter fracture with moderate symptoms was reported by Franey et al. (1988), who stated that 13 months after subclavian catheter implantation the patient

...noted a mild acute discomfort in the subclavian area while playing golf. Saline infusion into the device created pain and swelling in the same region and blood drawing was impossible. Chest X-ray revealed the device in place with one end of the catheter tip in the region of the subclavian vein and a separate segment of the catheter in the right atrium and ventricle. A nuclear medicine study using technetium-99 showed the proximal segment to be outside the vein. The catheter fragment was retrieved via a percutaneous right femoral vein approach using a snare. Examination of the 13.5 cm segment revealed a fish-mouth appearance at the point of fracture.

The report continued:

As described earlier it is the pinching force between the clavicle and first rib with any shoulder and pectoral girdle movement which causes the catheter to fracture. The patient involved in this case report is an avid golfer. Golf requires a great deal of shoulder and pectoral girdle motion to swing the club. It is this exact motion which is implicated in catheter failure.

Hinke et al. (1990) created a grading scale for the pinchoff syndrome (POS); grade 0 was used to designate no catheter narrowing. If the catheter exhibits bending from a smooth curve, grade 1 is used. Grade 2 identifies narrowing and grade 3 is used for transection and embolization. In a 6-year study of 987 implants using Silastic catheters, 11 met the foregoing criteria for the pinchoff syndrome within 3 weeks of catheter implantation. One patient exhibited grade 3 (fracturing and embolization); the others exhibited grade 1 or 2. The pinchoff incidence in this study was therefore 1.1%.

Bach et al. (1991) reported catheter fracture and extravasation, stating:

A 47-year-old woman had acute myeloid leukemia diagnosed in March 1988. The patient had a Port-a-Cath catheter (Pharmacia Deltec Inc., St. Paul, MN) implanted medially in the left infraclavicular region before chemotherapy. We inserted the catheter in the space between the clavicle and the first rib and passed it through the subclavian vein and vena cava superior to the entry of the right atrium.

The report continued:

Ten months later, during infusion of chemotherapy, the patient had paresthesia and severe pains in the left infraclavicular region and paresis of the left upper limb. The infusion was stopped immediately, but clinical evaluation showed no neurologic or cardiovascular deficits, and the symptoms disappeared within a few minutes. Radiography showed the catheter *in sutu*, but contrast injection confirmed our suspicion of catheter damage with leak of contrast in the area of the left costoclavicular ligament. We removed the catheter, and subsequent close examination demonstrated a weak, thin area with a large irregular fissure (incompatible with a cut during its original placement).

A similar catheter fracture was reported by Lafreniere (1991), who stated that in November 1988:

A Port-A-Cath was also inserted in the right subclavian vein using a percutaneous technique. A chest X-ray obtained post-operatively confirmed proper positioning of the catheter. Post-operatively, she was placed on high-dose folinic acid and 5-fluorouracil (5-FU) given at monthly intervals until October 1989 when an attempt at flushing her Port-A-Cath created intense pain along the course of the subcutaneous catheter. A chest X-ray done at that time revealed that the catheter had fractured at the junction of the first rib and clavicle and that the distal segment had embolized into the right atrium. The embolized segment was easily removed percutaneously through the right femoral vein; 2 weeks later a new Port-A-Cath was inserted in the left subclavian vein and removal of the right venous access was also carried out. Examination of the tip of the catheter disclosed pattern consistent with a fracture secondary to mechanical shearing forces associated with a compressed fish-mouth appearance at the fracture site.

Lafreniere (1991) reviewed the literature and uncovered 13 additional cases of subclavian catheter fracture; all catheters were used for chemotherapy. On viewing these cases and his own experience, he provided the following recommendations:

1) The subclavian puncture should be made at the mid-clavicular location rather than more medially; 2) fluoroscopic assessment at the time of insertion and a chest X-ray in the upright position would be done to look for catheter kinking; 3) if kinking is identified then a chest X-ray at 2 monthly intervals should be done to identify progression of kinking; 4) if any evidence of kinking is seen on follow-up chest X-ray, the catheter should probably be removed before 6 months has elapsed, as the mean time to fracture in this review was 6.5 months, and then replaced if necessary with another catheter.

The foregoing cases illustrate several types of catheter mishaps, identifying the symptoms and offering an explanation for their occurrence. It is to be pointed out that catheter electrodes are also subject to pinchoff and can be damaged.

CONDUCTING PROPERTIES OF FLUID-FILLED CATHETERS

Modern catheters are made of plastic, which is a good electrical insulator. However, such catheters are usually fluid filled, often with 0.9% saline. Radioopaque solutions and intravenous fluid, such as whole blood, plasma, 5% dextrose in water (D5W), urine, and bile, may also be transported by catheters. Most of these fluids, except D5W, are fairly good conductors of electric current. The electrical resistance (R) of a fluid-filled catheter depends on the length (L), inversely on the cross-sectional area (A) of the catheter, and directly with the resistivity (ρ) of the fluid therein. The resistance R = ρL/A, where R is in ohms, L and A are in centimeter units, and ρ in ohm-cm; Table 1 lists the resistivity values for several body fluids and those often carried by catheters. Radioopaque (contrast) medium may be a good or poor conductor and is available in two types, ionic and nonionic, the latter having a higher resistivity than the former. The nonionic types were developed to minimize the sensation felt when injected intravascularly.

Monsees and McQuarrie (1971) investigated the resistance of fluid-filled catheters with a view toward identifying whether they constituted a low- or high-resistance path into the body. Using resistivity values of 80 and 130 Ω-cm for physiological saline and blood, respectively, the resistance of a typical cardiac catheter can be calculated. For example, an 8F catheter has an internal diameter of 1.42 mm; for a 100-cm length, the resistances when filled with saline and blood are 0.5 and 0.8 MΩ, respectively. In other words, these two examples chosen illustrate that the resistance is quite high.

It should be noted that if the tip of a fluid-filled catheter is in contact with the myocardium, it is possible to calculate the voltage required to induce ventricular fibrillation. For example, many studies have shown (see Geddes and Baker 1989) that 50 μA rms of 60 Hz applied for about a few seconds will induce ventricular fibrillation. Therefore, the voltage needed to obtain this current is the product of this current and the resistance. For the 0.5- and 0.8-MΩ fluid-filled catheters, the rms voltages are 25 and 40. If the catheter tip is not against the endocardium, a higher voltage would be needed to produce fibrillation. It should be noted that the voltage would be much lower for a catheter electrode with 1000-ohm impedance. In this case, ventricular fibrillation would be produced by 50 mV. Calculations can be made for fluid-filled catheters of other diameters and lengths using the data in Tables 1 and 2, the latter providing the internal diameters of catheters. Note that for the French (F) scale, the outer diameter in millimeters is the F size divided by three.

CATHETER ELECTRODE PINCHOFF

Catheter-borne electrodes are placed in the heart via a venous route for pacing, cardioversion, and defibrillation. A catheter may carry a single electrode and a single conductor (monopolar) or it may carry two conductors connected to two electrodes (bipolar). Some catheters carry electrodes to stimulate both the atria and ventricles. In such a case there could be two, three, or four conductors in the catheter. Damage to such electrode catheters could allow the entry of tissue fluids leading to current escape and shunting, as well as corrosion. In such a case, sensing and/or pacing could be impaired. Malfunction could consist of conductor breakage or short circuit.

Stokes et al. (1987) reported that since 1980, nearly 5000 explanted pacemakers were examined, and of them, 1.8% exhibited fractured leads, the fracture being located 27 ± 5 cm from the terminal pin. They stated that lead failure occurred due to crushing and that the fracture was located at the point "where the lead crosses the first rib in very close approximation to the sterno-clavicular joint." In a subsequent paper, Stokes and McVenes (1988) stated that: "The fracture could be attributed to clamping between the first rib and clavicle."

TABLE 1
Resistivity of Fluids

Fluid Type	Temperature (°C)	Resistivity (ohm-cm)
Blood (40%)	37	130
Plasma	37	53
Saline (0.9%)	37	60
Saline (0.9%)	25	80
CSF	25	65
Bile	37	60
Amniotic fluid	37	50
Urine	37	30
Whole milk (cow)	35	170
D5W	Room	67,000
Radioopaque fluids		
Potassium iodide		
5%	Room	30
10%	Room	15
Hypaqueand[b] (50%)	Room	70
Omnipaque[b] (180 mg/Ml)	Room	1,857
Ioxilan[c] (300 mg/ml)	Room	4,500

[a] Resistivity increases with decreasing temperature, typically 2%/°C.

[b] Sanofi-Winthrop.

[c] Cook Imaging.

TABLE 2
Catheter Dimensions

Catheter Size "F"	Thick-Walled Catheter		Thin-Walled Catheter	
	Outer Diameter (mm)	Lumen Diameter (mm)	Outer Diameter (mm)	Lumen Diameter (mm)
3F	1.00	0.36	—	—
4F	1.33	0.46	1.33	0.58
5F	1.67	0.66	1.67	0.86
6F	2.00	0.91	2.00	1.17
7F	2.33	1.17	2.33	1.47
8F	2.67	1.42	2.67	1.73
9F	3.00	1.63	3.00	1.98
10F	3.33	1.83	3.33	2.24
11F	3.67	2.11	3.67	2.49
12F	4.00	2.39	4.00	2.74
14F	4.67	2.90	4.67	3.25

From catalog of the U.S. Catheter & Instrument Company, Glens Falls, NY.

Stokes and McVenes reported that pacing catheter damage can manifest itself in many ways, stating:

> Silicone rubber leads with parallel bipolar conductors can have the insulation between coils cut through due to external pressure. Some coaxial leads have outer coils fractured by a crushing mechanism. Some unipolar leads have exhibited flattened spots on the conductors, coil fracture due to fatigue and/or insulation failure.

Jacobs et al. (1993) called attention to the difference between flexural and compression (pinchoff) fracture in pacemaker leads. They found that the compression fracture was located 27.5 ± 5.2 cm distal to the connector pin on a 58-cm lead. The average time to failure was 11.1 months, with a range of 1 day to 53 months. They estimated the average incidence of such fractures was 1 to 2%. In addition to these studies they performed an experiment in a cadaver in which pressure in a balloon catheter in the subclavian vein was measured for different arm positions and different balloon sites. They stated:

> It was demonstrated fluoroscopically that in some instances kinking of the balloon catheter with these (arm) motions was causing pressure changes. There was little evidence fluoroscopically of any compressive effect at the costoclavicular angle from these motions. With caudal traction, however, there was compression that could be identified fluoroscopically with medially and laterally placed catheters. Significantly higher pressures were generated with caudal traction in the medially placed catheters with a mean of 126 ± 26 mmHg change from baseline compared to 63 ± 15 mmHg change for laterally placed catheters and 38 ± 13 mmHg change for catheters placed through the cephalic vein (P < 0.01).

From the studies on the explanted leads and those on the cadavers, they concluded:

> Our data suggest that it would be preferable to avoid the costoclavicular angle completely, either by placing the lead percutaneously into the axillary vein lateral to the costoclavicular ligamentous complex or by insertion through the cephalic vein. Most described techniques of subclavian venipuncture in the literature use landmarks that directly traverse the medial costoclavicular angle. Laterally the vein is more difficult to cannulate and injury to the subclavian artery and brachial plexus is potentially more problematic.

A different view of the cause of catheter fracture was presented by Magney et al. (1993), who performed catheter implant studies on cadavers. Careful dissections were then used to determine the path taken by the catheter electrode. They concluded:

> While blood vessels can be compressed by movements of the clavicle, our research suggests that lead and catheter damage in that region is caused by soft tissue entrapment rather than bony contact.

Magney et al. (1993) concluded by stating:

The placement of the lead should be checked by multiview cineradiography during movements of the ipsilateral upper extremity to ensure that leads or catheters have not been entrapped by the subclavius muscle or the costoclavicular ligament. If cineradiography is not available, posteroanterior chest X-rays (as described) should be used to confirm that newly placed leads are free of soft tissue entrapment.

CURRENT SINKS AND SOURCES

A medical device connected to a patient can function as a return path (sink) or as a provider (source) of current that can do harm. When a catheter or electrodes are applied to a subject, there is the opportunity for undesired current flow and whether or not it does harm depends on the local current density and duration of current flow.

An example of a medical device acting as a current sink is shown in Figure 2. A patient is connected to a grounded (G) medical device via an intravascular catheter, the fluid in which is in contact with ground via the device. An electrosurgical unit (ESU) is used to cut and/or coagulate tissue of the patient via an active electrode. However, the return conductor from the dispersive electrode to the ESU is interrupted at X. Therefore, on activating the ESU, the return path for the electrosurgical current is via the distributed capacitance (C) of the ESU to ground and via the intravascular catheter to ground (G) through the medical device. If, instead of a catheter, recording electrodes were on the patient, they could constitute the return path for the electro-surgical current. These undesired current routes are known as alternate current paths and if adequate ESU current flows, thermal injury can result at the point of contact with the patient.

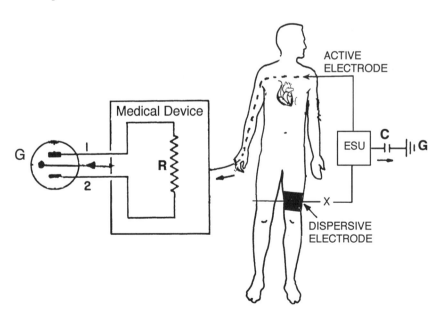

FIGURE 2 Current flow through a catheterized, grounded (G) subject as a result of inter-ruption (X) of the return path to the electrosurgical unit (ESU).

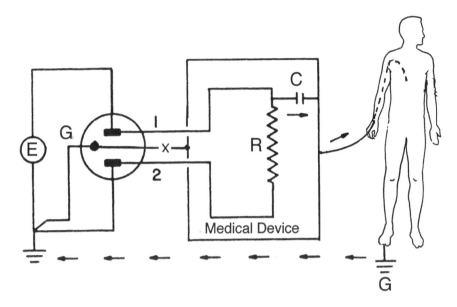

FIGURE 3 Leakage current caused to flow through a grounded subject via an intravascular catheter by interrupting (X) the conductor that grounds (G) the metal case of the device.

Figure 3 illustrates the situation in which the medical device acts as a source of current flowing through an intravascular catheter to a grounded (G) patient. The source of the (leakage) current is from the hot side of the power line (1), through the distributed capacitance (C) in the medical device. This current is present because the conductor that grounds the medical device is interrupted at X. If the leakage current is large enough, ventricular fibrillation can result. However, if the connection to ground were not interrupted at X, no leakage current would flow through the subject.

ELECTROSURGICALLY -INDUCED VENTRICULAR FIBRILLATION WITH FLUID-FILLED CATHETERS

Electrosurgical current can stimulate nerve, skeletal, and cardiac muscle. Therefore, it follows that it can produce ventricular fibrillation. The first report of such an event in man was presented by Hungerbuhler and Swope (1974); the report states:

> A 24-year-old woman was scheduled for elective surgical correction of an asymptomatic secondum-type atrial septal defect. Preoperatively, a central venous catheter and two intravenous catheters were inserted percutaneously. A left radial arterial catheter connected to an electronic pressure transducer (Hewlett-Packard) was also inserted. An electrocardiographic oscilloscope, with an electrocardiographic pad placed under the back, was used. An additional electrocardiogram was monitored with extremity leads connected to a system designed for amplification of low-level electronic signals originating within the body. A patient grounding plate was placed under the right buttock; the ground clip was attached and then plugged into the electrosurgical unit.

During the initial part of the surgery, the electrocautery was used to cauterize bleeding vessels in the subcutaneous fat, which resulted in the usual amount of high-frequency interference on the oscilloscope. The auscultatory esophageal rhythm remained regular.

However, 5 to 10 seconds after application of the electrosurgical knife in the cutting mode to the sternal periosteum, the auscultatory rhythm was noted to be irregular and then absent. Simultaneously, an increased electrical high-frequency interference appeared on the electrocardiographic oscilloscope. When the high-frequency interference cleared, the patient was noted to be in ventricular fibrillation, and had a blood pressure of less than 50 mmHg systolic.

The patient was immediately resuscitated over the next 70 seconds with external cardiac massage, lidocaine (150 mg total intravenous dose), phenylephrine (Neosynephrine) hydrochloride (2 mg given intravenously), and direct-current electroshock (200 watt-seconds) with paddles applied to the thorax.

The patient recovered and later it was found that the ground clip to the ground plate was disconnected and examined. A paper remnant torn from a previously used disposable ground plate was discovered wedged into the clip, but contact appeared adequate. Further, the male ground plug to the unit itself was noted to be loose. The unit was replaced with another electrosurgical unit (the same model) with the same ground plate and a new clip.

Electrosurgically induced ventricular fibrillation had been reported on the dog by Becker et al. (1974). Geddes et al. (1975) and Geddes (1979) produced ventricular fibrillation in the dog in which a saline-filled catheter in the right ventricle was connected to a blood-pressure transducer. A dispersive electrode was placed under the dog in dorsal recumbency. The active electrode was used to cut the skin prior to a thoracotomy and no cardiac arrhythmia occurred. The dispersive electrode was then disconnected and ESU current was delivered to the active electrode applied to the chest, and ventricular fibrillation occurred.

In the foregoing cases, the subject and the associated recording devices were a sink for the electrosurgical current. The arrows in Figures 2 and 3 illustrate the current paths.

An explanation for the induction of ventricular fibrillation with electrosurgical current was presented by Foster and Geddes (1986). It was shown that the presence of an arc at the active-electrode/tissue interface produces pulsating current that causes stimulation. It had been shown by Pearce (1986) and Tucker et al. (1984) that the presence of an arc in the path of electrosurgical current alters the frequency spectrum markedly, producing low-frequency components capable of stimulation.

60-Hz LEAKAGE CURRENT -INDUCED VENTRICULAR FIBRILLATION

Leakage current is an undesired current passing through a subject connected to a power-line-operated medical device. In this case the device is the current source. The effect of leakage current depends on its magnitude, pathway, and the duration of flow. Safe 60-Hz current limits and different types of patient contact have been established by AAMI (1978), along with the methods of testing devices for leakage current.

By far, the most hazardous leakage current is that borne by intravascular catheters. Figure 3 illustrates how leakage current due to distributed capacitance (C) within an ungrounded medical device allows power-line (60-Hz) current to flow through a cardiac catheterized subject who is grounded (G). The current is caused to flow by an interruption (X) in the connection that grounds the case of the device by its connection to the grounding pin (G) of the three-prong plug (1,2). Note that one side (2) of the 117-V (E) power line is grounded; this is typically done where the power line enters into the building.

Medical devices can malfunction and send enough current through a patient to do harm. The following examples illustrate this point. Such events were very common in the 1960s; they are less common today because of the performance requirements imposed by the FDA and compliance with applicable AAMI/ANSI standards.

Ventricular fibrillation due to leakage current from a densitometer connected to a cardiac catheter was reported by Mody et al. (1962). With the catheter tip at different sites, blood was drawn into the densitometer to measure oxygen saturation. Mody et al. reported:

> Pressures and blood-oxygen saturations were obtained from the right pulmonary artery, the main pulmonary artery, the outflow tract, and the cavity of the right ventricle. The tip of the catheter was then withdrawn into the right atrium so that its blood-oxygen saturation could be estimated. At precisely that instant the technician operating the instrument received an electric shock, and the patient began to show convulsive movements of the body and limbs. The catheter was immediately disconnected from the densitometer and withdrawn until the tip was in the superior vena cava. The electrocardiograph showed ventricular fibrillation, and the patient had become unconscious and was not breathing.

The patient was ultimately resuscitated and Mody et al. investigated the accident, stating:

> Our patient suffered the effects of direct electrical stimulation of the myocardium through the saline contents of a cardiac catheter connected to a Colson densitometer. The densitometer had previously been used without ill effects and in precisely the same manner for blood-oxygen sampling from the pulmonary artery and right ventricle. At the time of sampling from the right atrium, movement of the apparatus may have resulted in loss of contact of the earth (ground) lead from the densitometer, thereby allowing a current to flow from the chassis of the apparatus through the catheter into the patient.

Clearly this is a case in which the medical device (densitometer) was the source of the current, as illustrated in Figure 3.

A case of ventricular fibrillation due to catheter-borne leakage current was reported by Bousvaros et al. (1962) at a time when many medical devices exhibited a relatively high leakage current. They reported:

> A No. 8 N.I.H. catheter was introduced into the right ventricle for cine-angiographic studies of the right ventricular outflow tract and pulmonary valve.

When, by the use of the fluoroscope, the tip of the catheter was seen to lie in the region of the apex of the right ventricle, the catheter was connected to a Gidlund high-power injection syringe. At the moment of connection, considerable interference developed in the electrocardiographic tracing on the oscilloscope, implying a change in the electrical environment of the patient. Owing to this interference, it was not possible to read the electrocardiogram, but within a few seconds it was noted that the patient had become rigid, and on the fluoroscope the heart was seen to be fibrillating. The injector was disconnected; immediately the interference stopped and the ventricular fibrillation was noted on the electrocardiogram. Open-heart cardiac massage was performed immediately, and after three shocks were applied to the surface of the heart with an internal defibrillator, normal rhythm was restored.

Subsequent investigation of this accident revealed that the patient was grounded via the EKG electrodes and that the electrically driven power injector was inadequately grounded. They stated that it was the contrast agent in the catheter that carried the current to the heart. Commenting on the conductivity of the contrast agent, they stated: "furthermore, it was found that 50% diatrizoate solution was a somewhat better conductor than either saline or blood." In this accident, the medical device (injector) was the source of the current.

In addition to ventricular fibrillation due to leakage current flowing through a contrast-medium filled cardiac catheter, Viamonte and Hobbs (1967) pointed out earlier that the same event can be induced by the sudden injection of contrast agent into a ventricle; they stated: "ventricular fibrillation may be triggered by the injection of contrast material against the surface of the heart during the vulnerable period of ventricular repolarization."

The vulnerable period is that time during recovery of the ventricles when a single stimulus will precipitate ventricular fibrillation. The center of this period is associated with the T wave of the ECG (Jones and Geddes, 1977).

Rowe and Zarnstorff (1965) commented on the possibility of ventricular fibrillation resulting from contrast agent striking the endocardium during the vulnerable period; they stated:

> The endocardial stimulation provided by forcible ejection of contrast material against its surface is enough to provoke ventricular premature contractions in most subjects during intraventricular injection. Presumably this stimulus could occur in the vulnerable period of ventricular repolarization.

Rowe and Zarnstorff (1965) reported seven episodes of ventricular fibrillation in patients undergoing cineangiocardiography; these episodes were unrelated to grounding of the electromechanical injector or to contrast agent striking the endocardium. A solenoid-driven injector was used and it was noted that the onset of fibrillation was associated with opening of the injector switch. They documented the source of the electrical transient that induced fibrillation and stated:

> It was demonstrated that each time the injector switch was released (opened), an electrical discharge of 40 V was delivered for 1 to 2 msec to the syringe in the injector. A smaller and more variable transient occurred when the circuit was closed.

Furthermore, during opening and closing of the injector switch, transients could be demonstrated on the oscilloscopic tracing of the ECG of a dog attached to the injector by a cardiac catheter filled with contrast substance. A similar injector from another hospital produced the same type of electrical discharge, as did an injector manufactured by another company. (Their paper describes a simple circuit for eliminating this transient.)

REFERENCES

AAMI — Association for the Advancement of Medical Instrumentation. Safe current limits for electromedical apparatus (1978). AAMI. 330 Washington Blvd., Arlington, VA 22201-4598.

Aitken, D.R. and Minton, J.P. The pinch-off sign. *Am. J. Surg.* 1984, 148: 633–636.

Bach, F., Videbaek, C., Holst-Christensen, J., et al. Cystostatic extravasation. *Cancer* 1991, 68: 538–539.

Becker, C.M., Malhotra, I.V., and Hedley-White, J. The distribution of radio-frequency current and burns. *Anesthesiology* 1974, 38(2): 106–122.

Bousvaros, G.A., Dan, C., and Hopps, J.A. An electrical hazard of selective angiography. *Can. Med. Assn. J.,* 1962, 87: 286–288.

Foster, K.S. and Geddes, L.A. The cause of stimulation with electrosurgical current. *Med. Instrum.* 1986, 20(6): 335–336.

Frager, C. and Hertzberg, R. Spontaneous intravenous catheter fracture and embolization from an implanted venous access port and analyses by seaming electron microscopy. *Cancer* 1987, 60: 270–273.

Franey, T., De Marco, L.C., Geiss, A.C., et al. Catheter fracture and embolization in a totally implanted venous access catheter. *J. Paren. Enteral Nutrition* 1988, 12(5): 528–530.

Geddes, L.A. and Baker, L.E. *Principles of Applied Biomedical Instrumentation.* 1989. Wiley Interscience, New York.

Geddes, L.A., Tacker, W.A., and Cabler, P. A new electrical hazard associated with the electrocautery. *Med. Instrum.* 1975, 9(2): 112–113.

Geddes, L.A. Ventricular fibrillation due to low and high frequency electrical current. Proc. 14th AAMI Conf., 1979, 14: 88.

Groshong, L.E. and Brown, R.J. Valved Two-Way Catheter. U.S. Patent 4,549,879 (October 29, 1985) and 4,671,796 (June 9, 1987).

Hinke, D.H., Zandt-Stastny, D.A., Goodman, L.R., et al. Pinch-off syndrome. *Radiology* 1990, 177: 353–356

Hungerbuhler, R.F. and Swope, J.P. Ventricular fibrillation associated with the use of electrocautery. *J.A.M.A.* 1974, 230(3): 431–435.

Jacobs, D.M., Fink, A.S., Miller, R.P., et al. Anatomical and morphological evaluation of pacemaker lead compression. *PACE* 1993, 16: 434–444.

Jones, M. and Geddes, L.A. Strength-duration curves for acardiac pacemaking and ventricular fibrillation. *Cardiovascular Res. Center Bull.* 1977, 15: 101–112.

Lafreniere, R. Indwelling subclavian catheter and a visit with the pinchedoff sign. *J. Surg. Oncol.* 1991, 47: 261–264.

Magney, J.E., Flynn, D.M., Parsons, J.A., et al. Anatomical mechanisms explaining damage to pacemaker leads. *PACE* 1993, 16: 445–451.

Mody, S.M., Foona, M.B., and Richings, M. Ventricular fibrillation resulting from electrocution during cardiac catheterization. *Lancet* 1962, 2: 698–699.

Monsees, L.R. and McQuarrie, D.G. Is an intravascular catheter a conducer? *Med. Electron. Data* 1971, 12: 26–27.

Pearce, J.A. *Electrosurgery.* 1986. Chapman & Hall, London.

Prager, D. and Hertzberg, R.W. Spontaneous intravenous catheter fracture and embolization. Bancer. 1987, 60: 270–272.

Rowe, G. G. and Zarnstorff, W. G. Ventricular fibrillation during selective angiocardiography. *J.A.M.A.* 1965, 192(11): 105–108.

Stokes, K. and McVenes, R. Pacing lead fracture, a previously unknown complication of subclavian stick. Cardiostim 88,265 P/755. *PACE* 1988, 11: 855.

Stokes, K., Staffenson, D., Lesser, J., et al. A possible new complications of subclavian stick: conductor fracture. *PACE* 1987, Part II 10: 748.

Tucker, R.D., Schmitt, O.H., Silvert, C.E., and Silvis, S.E. Demodulated low frequency currents from electrosurgical procedures. *Surg. Gynecol. Obst.* 1984, 159: 39–43.

Viamonte, M. and Hobbs, J. Automatic electric injector. *Invest. Radiol.* 1967, July–August: 262–265.

6 Direct-Current Injury

CONTENTS

INTRODUCTION

Today there are only a few instances in which direct current is passed through living tissue intentionally; perhaps the best examples are for transdermal drug delivery (iontophoresis), bone-growth stimulation, fracture healing, and hair removal by electrolysis. In the last century, direct current was passed through the entire body and applied locally; the method was known as "galvanism" or "galvanotherapy", which was used to treat a variety of bizarre ailments (Geddes, 1983). Galvanopuncture was the term used when the direct current flowed through a needle inserted into the skin. At the needle tip, electrolysis and heating occurred; when the latter was used, the term "galvanocautery" was applied. This technique is used to make lesions of controlled size; Geddes (1972) reviewed the literature; electrolysis for permanent hair removal represents the modern application of galvanopuncture.

It is possible to estimate the size of the lesion produced by direct current injected by a needle electrode. Although most of the lesions studied were produced in animal brains, the results in other soft tissues are not expected to be very different. Most of the studies employed needle electrodes about 0.5 to 1 mm diameter insulated down to a small tip. Without regard to polarity (which is of some importance in the studies that were performed carefully), the range of current multiplied by time varies between 20 to about 90 mA-sec; these parameters produced spherical lesions having diameters of about 1 to 1 1/2 mm. There is ample evidence that with high currents (i.e., greater than about 5 mA) and long times (in the range of minutes), the lesion diameter is not proportional to the product of milliamperes and seconds. Lesions with flat plate electrodes will be larger than the extent of the plate and the severity of the injury will be the greatest under the perimeter of the electrode where the current density is highest (Caruso et al., 1979, and Overmeyer et al., 1979).

165

Consider a pair of electrodes placed on tissue and direct current is passed. Electrolysis of tissue fluids occurs with low current density. At the cathode, the tissues will become acidic due to the accumulation of hydrogen ions (H^+). At the anode, the tissues will become basic due to the accumulation of hydroxyl (OH^-) ions. Other electrolytic products will also be liberated such as oxygen, chlorine, sodium, etc. If the current density is high, heating will occur and first-, second-, or third-degree burns can result. Such lesions are painful and slow to heal.

If the direct current is applied suddenly, sensory receptors and motor nerves will be stimulated. During constant current flow there should be no sensation, theoretically. However, due to the electrolysis, the current flow is not constant and a tingling sensation is usually perceived. If the current is interrupted suddenly, sensory and motor nerves can be stimulated.

IONTOPHORESIS

Iontophoresis is the term used when a direct current is applied to facilitate delivery of a soluble substance through the skin. When such a substance is placed on the skin, it will be absorbed, the rate of absorption being proportional to the difference in concentration of the substance and that of it in the skin. Initially, the concentration below the skin is zero, and with the passage of time the concentration rises and the transdermal concentration difference decreases, thereby reducing the rate of substance transport; this is Fick's law of diffusion. If the capillary blood flow removes the subdermal substance, it will continue to be absorbed. In the late 1800s it was discovered that the application of direct current to an electrode placed over a drug-coated skin site facilitated the transdermal transport of the drug.

The method of applying iontophoresis is shown in Figure 1, in which the drug to be transported is contained in a skin-surface (active) electrode (A) within which is an inert metal electrode that establishes electrolytic contact with the drug solution. The other inert (dispersive) electrode (B) is much larger in area and at a convenient distant site. Between the two electrodes is connected a constant direct-current source. The polarity is selected on the basis of the polarity of the charge on the drug molecule. For example, if the drug carries a positive charge, the active electrode is made positive. The opposite polarity is used if the charge on the drug molecule is negative. The pH of the solution in the active electrode chamber is important for efficient drug transport.

To avoid producing an unpleasant sensation, the current density (mA/cm^2) under the active electrode is kept low and the current is increased slowly to its selected value to avoid sensation. Likewise, when the treatment is to be terminated, the current is slowly reduced to zero before the electrodes are removed. If the current is turned on or off suddenly, the subject may feel a sensation like a pin prick, or stronger if the current density is high.

The amount of drug transported through the skin by iontophoresis depends on the current, its duration of flow, and the concentration of the drug in the active electrode chamber, as well as the pH. Treatment times usually last from 10 to 30 min. Currents up to 10 mA have been used and the treatment is quantitated in terms

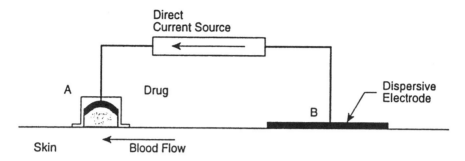

FIGURE 1   Principle of iontophoresis in which a constant direct current is used to transport drug molecules in an electrode chamber (A) into the skin. The return path for the current is via a large-area, dispersive electrode (B).

of charge, i.e., the product of milliamperes and minutes. The current density is usually much less than 1 mA/cm^2. High current density will produce an unpleasant pricking sensation.

COMPLICATIONS WITH IONTOPHORESIS

Apart from the use of excessive current which can produce an unpleasant skin sensation, there can be side effects due to the species of metal used in the active electrode chamber. Many different metals have been used for the active electrode which can be either positive or negative, depending on the charge on the drug molecule. Silver, tin, zinc, stainless steel, copper, and carbon-loaded silicone rubber have all been used. Because direct current is used, a wide variety of electrolytic products can be produced at the active electrode. For example, if silver is used and made positive, it is chlorided; if it is made negative, silver ions are transported into the skin producing a black spot. The presence of silver in the skin is called argyria. Copper ions have been intentionally deposited in the skin for their germicidal effect. Such heavy metal ions combine with proteins. For iontophoresis, it is wise to use an inert electrode material, such as stainless steel, platinum, gold, or carbon, and keep the current below the sensation threshold to avoid pain and skin sloughing.

DIRECT-CURRENT INJURIES

Injury from direct current usually results from device malfunction, misuse, or a design defect. In the following examples the injuries were not noticed because the patients were anesthetized and draped.

A direct-current injury investigated by the author involved an anesthetized patient who was prepared for surgery with two stimulating electrodes behind the knee and recording electrodes on the scalp to detect somatosensory-evoked potentials (SSEPs) during surgery. The patient was draped and the equipment was connected to the electrodes. During surgery, the equipment functioned normally. However, somehow the stimulating electrode cable became disconnected from the stimulator.

The electrodes were reconnected, not to the stimulus output, but to the battery-test jacks which were connected to an internal 90-V battery. The SSEPs were no longer recordable and at the end of the operation, when the patient was being prepared for transport to the ward, a very large electrochemical "burn" was found at the site of the two stimulating electrodes.

Tests carried out later with the stimulating electrodes placed on a thick slice of steak and connected to the battery-test jacks confirmed the possibility that the injury could have occurred this way. It was also argued that the injury was due to electrosurgical current, but this was not proven.

The foregoing case raises several important questions. For example, was the accident due to a lack of training of the technician who reconnected the stimulating electrodes? Did the stimulator have a design defect that allowed this inappropriate connection to be made? Finally, could this accident have been foreseen in terms of the possibility of connecting the stimulating electrodes to the battery-test jacks?

Leming et al. (1971) reported the following case of an electrochemical burn by low-voltage direct current; they stated:

A forty-year old white female underwent surgery which lasted 2 h. Before and during the administration of anesthesia, the patient was monitored with a cardioscope attached via four limb leads and a finger plethysmograph, the only electrical or electronic devices used throughout the procedure. Before the onset of anesthesia, the patient complained of a painful "pricking" sensation on the back of her left thumb, the finger to which the plethysmograph had been connected. The patient was reassured and put to sleep for the procedure. On the following day, in response to pain on the left thumb, examination revealed that the skin, which had been under the right leg electrode (the ECG ground lead), had multiple, discrete, punctate lesions not present before the operation. On the left thumb near the base of the fingernail, there was a dark gray, dry necrotic lesion with a small perforation near the center. On investigation, it was found that the 10-volt, direct current supply within the photo-plethysmograph resulted in a 10-volt potential difference between the right-leg (ground) ECG electrode and the plethysmograph case.

Leming et al. (1970) pointed out that "two ordinary flash-light batteries, for example, would not be classified as harmless, but accidental or intentional long-term contact with these devices will result in burn, especially if connected to devices in ohmic contact with a subject." Note that the voltage of two ordinary flashlight batteries is $2 \times 1.5 = 3$ V.

TERMINOLOGY

The term "burn" is often used to describe the lesions produced by direct current. The same term is used to describe chemically-induced lesions. This practice has arisen perhaps because it is convenient to use the burn scale (1st, 2nd, 3rd degree) to describe the lesions. A 1st-degree burn is skin reddening; a 2nd-degree burn is characterized by blisters. A 3rd-degree burn is a full skin-thickness lesion.

REFERENCES

Caruso, P., Pearce, J.A., and DeWitt, D.P. Temperature and current density distributions at electrosurgical dispersive electrode sites. *Proc. 7th N. Engl. Bioeng. Conf.* 1979, 373–374.

Geddes, L.A. *Electrodes and the Measurement of Bioelectric Events.* 1972. John Wiley & Sons, New York.

Geddes, L.A. A short history of the electrical stimulation of excitable tissue, including electrotherapeutic applications. *Physiologist* 1983, (Suppl.) 27(1): 1–47.

Leming, M.N., Jacob, R.G., and Howland, W.S. Low-voltage direct current plethysmograph burns. *Med. Res. Eng.* 1971, October–November: 19–21.

Leming, M.N., Ray, C., and Howland, W.S. Low-voltage, direct current burns. *J.A.M.A.* 1970, 30: 1681–1685.

Overmeyer, K., Pearce, J.A., and DeWitt, D.P. Measurements of temperature distribution at electrosurgical dispersive electrode sites. *Trans. ASME* 1979, 101: 66–72.

7 Transcutaneous Electrical Nerve Stimulation

CONTENTS

INTRODUCTION

Transcutaneous electrical nerve stimulation (TENS) employs mild, short-duration, repetitive electrical stimuli, applied to skin-surface electrodes to reduce or abolish acute or chronic pain, the latter being loosely defined as pain lasting more than 6 months. A TENS unit is prescribed by a physician and is operated by the patient. Because electrical stimuli are applied to the body, there is the possibility of such signals interfering with the operation of implanted electronic therapeutic devices.

TENS is used widely to relieve the pain associated with athletic injuries, trauma, surgical procedures, cancer, and childbirth. Among other conditions now treated are migraine, bursitis, tennis elbow, tendonitis, rheumatoid arthritis, tinnitus, diabetic neuropathy, radiculopathies, carpal tunnel syndrome, shoulder-hand syndrome, osteoarthritis, sciatica, sinus headache, reflex sympathetic dystrophy, and hemiplegic pain. Pain intensity is graded on a scale of 0 (no pain) to 10 (incapacitating pain). Although pain from any cause is amenable to TENS treatment, not all subjects experience complete relief. The 0 to 10 pain scale is used to identify the relief, i.e., by a reduction in the scale number. Adequate relief is obtained by about 50% of the subjects. There are many who believe that the use of TENS plus an analgesic reduces the amount of drug needed to suppress pain.

There are a few contraindications for the use of TENS; for example, in patients with demand cardiac pacemakers, the pacemaker could be inhibited if it detects the TENS pulses; this controversial situation will be discussed later in this chapter. TENS should not be used for undiagnosed pain; nor should it be used if the current flowing between the electrodes is transcranial. The effect of transcranial current is discussed elsewhere in this chapter. TENS should not be used with electrodes around the eyes because phosphenes (light flashes in the visual field) may be perceived.

Another contraindication is the placement of electrodes on the neck over the carotid sinuses, vagus, or laryngeal nerves, stimulation of which could produce cardiac arrhythmias.

MECHANISMS OF PAIN INHIBITION

Wall and Sweet (1967) discovered that pain could be suppressed by electrical stimulation of large-diameter sensory nerve (A) fibers which verified the gate theory of Melzack and Wall (1965). Wall and Sweet carried out studies on eight patients using direct-nerve and transcutaneous electrical stimulation. They applied 0.1-msec rectangular wave stimuli with a frequency of 100/sec. Superficial nerves were stimulated using needle or wire electrodes — a needle or wire paired with a skin-surface electrode or two skin-surface electrodes. In each case, the stimulus intensity was increased until a tingling sensation was perceived by the patient. In general, 2 min of stimulation provided about 30 min. of pain relief.

A second mechanism of pain suppression by TENS involves the endogenous secretion of morphine-like substances (endorphins) from the periaqueductal region in the brain. Sjolund and Eriksson (1976, 1979) advanced this theory on the basis of blockade of pain suppression by naloxone, a drug that inhibits the analgesic effect of morphine, the most potent pain killer.

The goal of TENS is to stimulate large-diameter, sensory afferent nerve fibers only; therefore, short-duration pulses of current are used because the chronaxie of these nerve fibers is shorter than that for pain fibers. Figure 1 shows normalized strength-duration curves for sensory (A) and pain (C) nerve fibers. Note that the current required for stimulating pain fibers starts to rise for a pulse duration shorter than about 2 msec; whereas the threshold for sensory fibers rises for a pulse duration shorter than about 0.05 msec. Therefore, the use of a stimulus of this duration will minimally stimulate pain and maximally stimulate sensory fibers.

CURRENT-PULSECHARACTERISTICSOFTENSUNITS

Although repetitive short-duration pulses are employed with TENS, there are many ways of delivering these pulses. Low-frequency TENS employs 2 to 5/sec pulses and high-frequency TENS uses 80 to 140/sec pulses. Some TENS units deliver short bursts twice/second, while another mode employs rhythmic modulation of the pulse width. Finally, some TENS units employ a positive/negative (biphasic) wave. All modalities seek to produce a mild tingling sensation. Table 1 presents a compilation of output characteristics of 18 TENS units. Note that pulse rates available range from less than 1 to 285/sec and the pulse widths available range from 16 to 720 μsec.

THE STIMULATOR

An interesting hand-operated, batteryless stimulator is the Stimulator, which produces sensory stimuli with a high-voltage pulse that is generated when the patient presses on a plunger, as shown in Figure 2. The device is held between the first and second fingers and the thumb presses on the plunger, which causes an internal

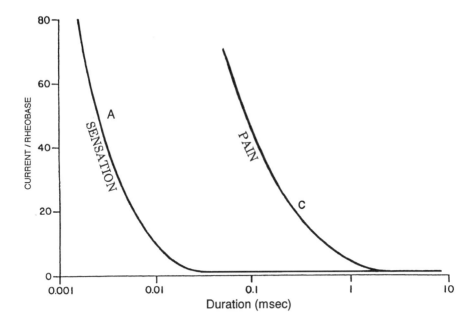

FIGURE 1 Normalized strength-duration curves for pain and sensation.

hammer to strike a piezoelectric crystal which, in turn, is connected to two concentric electrodes on the bottom of the device. The Stimulator is placed over the area of pain and the plunger is depressed, releasing a 40-kHz damped sinusoidal voltage pulse which produces the sensation. Note that the electrodes are dry and there are no batteries; the patient provides the mechanical energy that is converted to electrical energy. Multiple stimuli are used to reduce the pain. The same precautions as used with TENS units are applicable to the Stimulator.

ELECTRODE PLACEMENT

At present, there are no standard sites for TENS electrodes. Mannheimer (1978) and Mannheimer et al. (1978) recommended that the best sites were motor, acupuncture, and/or trigger points. A motor point is a skin site where the lowest stimulus intensity will evoke muscular contraction. A trigger point is a site where gentle pressure evokes a specific sensation, usually pain. In general, one electrode is placed over, or just proximal to, the site of pain and over a superficial nerve. The other electrode is placed distally at a convenient site. Uniform contact with the skin is essential to prevent the development of localized regions of high current density. Sometimes four electrodes are used with a two-channel TENS unit. Diagonal lines joining the electrodes form an X, the center of which is the pain site.

ELECTRODE TYPES

Two types of electrodes are used; one employs metal foil with a conductive gel and the other is black rubber or carbon-loaded silicone rubber. Usually any hair on the

TABLE 1
Output Characteristics of Typical TENS Units

Manufacturer	Rate/Sec	Amplitude mA PK-PK	Width μSEC	Charge μC Max/Pulse
A	7.1	41	200	3
B	2.9–131.6	130	60–140	19
C	2.3–106.4	480	200	100
D	0.9–87.7	110m	100–160	42
E	3.7–113.6	52	40–300	14
F	0.7–27.8	200	200	150
G	2.2–106.4	80	40–230	24
H	40.8–104	130	720	57
I	2–104.1	135	40–270	34
J	3.3–100	170	400	71
K	94.3b	120	150	59
L	2.1–192.3	78	50–600	41
M	14.300–14.3	8	34	0.14
N	1.8–119	160	45–120	23
O	4.2–151.5	70	50–250	16
P	2.2–50	230	350	71
Q	10.4–270	120	16–280	29
R	2.9–285	86	30–220	11

Note: b = bursts, m = modulated.
Data from *Health Devices,* June 1981. ECRI Plymouth Meeting, PA 19462.

skin site is clipped and the skin is washed with mild soap. After the electrodes are applied, the output of the TENS unit is increased very slowly until a mild tingling sensation is perceived. The relief of pain occurs slowly; often it requires more than 30 min to start to be perceived. Pain relief far outlasts cessation of stimulation.

STANDARDS OF PERFORMANCE

There is an AAMI/ANSI standard for the performance of TENS units. It sets performance requirements when the TENS unit is connected to a resistive load and specifies the maximum charge per pulse. The standard can be obtained from AAMI and is designated ANSI/AAMI — NS4-1985.

COMPLICATIONS WITH TENS UNITS

A TENS unit is a mild electrical stimulator, the output of which is set by the patient. For this reason only fully conscious, responsible patients should use a TENS unit. The patient must have been instructed on the proper use by a knowledgeable therapist.

Skin irritation accompanying the use of TENS has been reported by Zugerman (1982), who described a case of allergic contact dermatitis. It was found that the

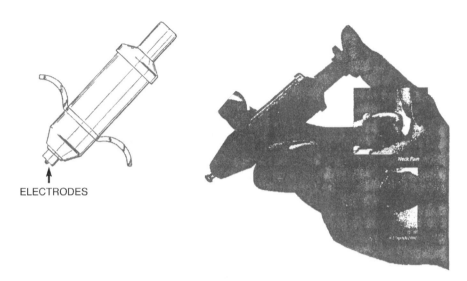

ELECTRODES

FIGURE 2   The Stimulator (A) and method of activating it (B) by holding it between the first and second fingers and depressing the plunger with the thumb. (Courtesy of Natural Innovations, Inc., Akron, OH 44319.)

conductive coupling agent used with the electrodes contained propylene glycol, to which the patient was allergic, verified by a patch test. Patch tests with other coupling agents revealed one that produced no irritation, and with it the patient was able to resume TENS treatments.

Bolton (1983) suggested that the skin reaction that Zugerman reported could be due to electrochemical decomposition of the conducting coupling medium at the electrode-skin surfaces where hydrogen and hydroxyl ions are liberated. While this can occur with unidirectional current pulses, the positive patch test with propylene glycol indicates that the patient was allergic to this chemical constituent of the electrode coupling medium.

To avoid skin reaction under TENS electrodes, Bolton (1983) recommended the use of a 1- to 2-mm-thick gauze pad, moistened thoroughly with physiological saline (0.9%) or weak buffer as the electrode coupling agent. She also recommended the use of a waveform consisting of a short train of positive-going pulses followed immediately by an identical train of negative-going pulses. In this way there is no net charge delivered and, hence, no net electrochemical decomposition of the coupling agent.

There has been some concern about the safety of TENS in obstetrics because the electrodes are close to the fetus *in utero*. Typically, the electrodes are placed on the lower back (T-10,11, S-2, 4) or the suprapubic region. Bundsen and Ericson (1982) reported that in over 500 obstetric patients undergoing TENS, no harmful effects have been observed in the mother or child.

The ability of a TENS unit to interfere with an implanted demand cardiac pacemaker is a controversial issue. Such a device senses the electrical activity of the heart and, if present, is inhibited. Such a pacemaker could sense low-frequency

TENS pulses and be inhibited. There is also the possibility of reprogramming of the pacemaker by TENS pulses. Whether or not these events occur depends on the type of pacemaker, the type of electrodes (monopolar or bipolar), the distance and orientation of the TENS electrodes with respect to the pacing lead, and the intensity and type of pulses delivered by the TENS unit. It should also be noted that implantable nerve and muscle stimulators are used for a variety of purposes and the output of such devices could be detected by a demand pacemaker or automatic cardioverter defibrillator. Whether there are few such incidents or whether many are unreported is not known.

Shade (1985) reported on her experience with a 74-year-old, 200-lb man with a cardiac pacemaker who had metastatic cancer and was using TENS to control pain. The TENS electrodes were placed on the left lateral chest, two slightly anteriorly and two posteriorly at the 5th and 10th intercostal areas. The amplitude range for this unit was 0 to 130 V, the frequency range 12 to 100/sec, and the pulse width range was 120 to 330 µsec. A stimulation pulse width of 20 µsec was used. The rate and amplitude were set at 5 to give a frequency of 35 pulses per second (pps). At this setting, the patient's pain was rated 2 vs. a maximal rating of 10 at pretreatment. This decrease in pain occurred within 1 h after TENS application. The patient used the TENS unit 24 h/day. Shade stated that "an ECG readout was taken before the TENS unit was applied that showed strong, sufficient cardiac rhythm. Once the TENS unit was applied, the settings were slowly increased to the level of pain relief. This increase was achieved with a rate of 35 pulses per second. During this adjustment period, continuous ECG readouts were taken for approximately two minutes." No cardiac arrhythmia was observed. She concluded by stating "with close monitoring, some patients may be able to wear a TENS unit simultaneously with cardiac pacemakers." Shade recommended recording the ECG while increasing the output of the TENS unit with pacemaker patients.

Rasmussen et al. (1988) applied TENS at four sites to 51 patients with 20 models of cardiac pacemakers. The sites were on the same side of the body as the pacemaker and included the lumbar, neck, left leg, and lower arm. The TENS frequency was 24.7/sec and no episodes of interference or reprogramming were encountered. They stated:

> We believe that most patients with permanent cardiac pacemakers can safely undergo TENS. We suggest that the TENS electrodes not be placed parallel to the pacemaker electrode vector until studies have verified the safety of this positioning.

This admonition is very relevant because if the TENS electrodes are on the chest in a line parallel to the pacemaker electrode axis, there will be the maximum likelihood of the pacemaker sensing the TENS pulses.

When considering the possibility of a TENS unit interfering with a demand cardiac pacemaker, it is important to distinguish between low-frequency and high-frequency TENS. The former employs 2 to 5 pulses/sec, which is equivalent to 120 to 300/min, which is in the heart-rate range. Because the sensing circuits in demand pacemakers are band-pass limited, high-frequency TENS may not be so easily detected as low-frequency TENS.

REFERENCES

AAMI — Association for the Advancement of Medical Instrumentation. 3330 Washington Blvd. Suite, 400, Arlington, VA 22201-4598.

Bolton, L. TENS electrode irritation. *J. Am. Acad. Dermatol.* 1983, 8: 134–135.

Bundsen, P. and Ericson, L. Pain relief in labor by TENS. *Acta Obst. Gynecol. Scand.* 1982, 61: 1–5.

Health Devices. Emergency Care Research Institute, 5200 Butler Pike, Plymouth Meeting, PA 19462.

Mannheimer, G.S. Electrode placement for transcutaneous electrical nerve stimulation. *Phys. Therapy* 1978, 58(12): 1455–1462.

Mannheimer, G.S. et al. *Clinical Transcutaneous Electrical Nerve Stimulation.* 1978. Davis, Philadelphia.

Melzack, R. and Wall, P.D. Pain mechanisms: a new theory. *Science* 1965, 150: 971–979.

Rasmussen, M.J., Hayes, D.L., and Vlietstra, R.E. Can transcutaneous electrical nerve stimulation be safely used in patients with permanent cardiac pacemakers? *Proc. Mayo Clin.* 1988, 63(5): 443–445.

Shade, S.K. Transcutaneous electrical nerve stimulation for a patient with a cardiac pacemaker. *Phys. Therapy* 1985, 65(2): 206–208.

Sjolund, B. and Eriksson, M. Electro-acupuncture and endogenous morphines. *Lancet* 1976, 11: 1085.

Sjolund, B. and Ericksson, M.B. Endorphins and analgesia produced by peripheral conditioning stimulation. *Advances in Pain Research and Therapy.* Bonica, J.J., Ed. 1979. Raven Press, New York.

Wall, P.D. and Sweet, W.H. Tempory abolition of pain in man. *Science* 1967, January 6: 108–109.

Zugerman, C. Dermatitis from transcutaneous electric nerve stimulation. *J. Am. Acad. Dermatol.* 1982, 6: 936–939.

8 Tissue Injury

CONTENTS

INTRODUCTION

There are many ways that living tissue can be injured in a medical environment. For example, thermal injury can be caused by coming into contact with heated objects; such accidents are discussed in the chapter on anesthesia. Thermal injury can be induced electrically by radiofrequency current; such accidents are described in the chapter on electrosurgery. Burn specialists distinguish between a thermal contact burn and an electrical burn. With the former, the heat is conducted from the heated object on the skin surface to the underlying tissue. The damage depends on the temperature of the heated object, its size, and how long it is in contact. The blanch test (see below) is often used to assess the subcutaneous capillary circulation which, if compromised, will cause the burn to become more prominent over a period of days.

With an electrical burn, the skin is actively heated by the current flow. The skin damage is usually apparent immediately. However, the subcutaneous tissues are also actively heated by the current and the damage depends on the current density (squared), the duration of current flow, and the resistivity of the tissues carrying the current. Electrosurgical burns are quite common when the dispersive electrode makes only partial contact with the skin. The relationship between the burn severity and the energy-density factor is discussed in the chapter on electrosurgery. Although an electrosurgical burn is usually evident immediately, if the subcutaneous capillaries are damaged, the lesion will become more evident with the passage of time.

With tissue injury, the term "burn treachery" is sometimes used and refers to the difficulty in predicting the future course of tissue damage. When skin is injured by coming into contact with a heated object, the superficial circulation is assessed by the blanch test, i.e., thumb pressure is applied, then released. If the tissue blanches and then reddens, this is evidence of circulation. If neither blanching nor reddening occurs, this is evidence that there is little or no local circulation and the underlying tissues will die, and the injury will become more apparent with the passage of time.

Direct current can also cause injury by heat and/or electrolysis; such accidents are discussed in the chapter on direct-current injury. Tissue can be injured by inadequate blood supply (ischemia). Prolonged lying or sitting in place compromises blood flow in the supported region, resulting in pressure sores; such events are described in this chapter. Pressure sores are rarely obvious at the time of insult, although very careful examination may reveal a blanched area. Pressure sores develop and may take a day or so to become apparent. Finally, tissues can be injured by chemical compounds; in such cases it is necessary to distinguish between injury due to the species of chemical and injury due to an allergic response. Both types are discussed in this chapter. Parenthetically, in describing allergic injuries, the thermal burn scale is used frequently. A first-degree burn is characterized by reddening (erythema). A second-degree burn is characterized by blisters and a third-degree burn is a full skin-thickness injury.

ISCHEMIC INJURY

Ischemia pertains to a deficiency of blood flow, the consequence of which depends on the particular tissue bed that is compromised. Tissue ischemia can result from the manner in which the body is supported, e.g., lying on an operating table or a bed or sitting in a chair for a prolonged period without moving. The tissue capillaries in the supporting region are compressed, thereby impeding blood flow. Typically, capillary pressure is about 30 mmHg. Pearce (1971, 1986) stated that hospital beds and surgical tables exert contact pressures between the patient and the table frequently in excess of 200 mmHg under the head, scapula, sacrum, heels, elbows, and the calf muscle (Babbs et al., 1990). In these typical locations, decubitus (lying down) ulcers are found most frequently over bony prominences. The places of highest contact pressure vary with the build of the person.

Figure 1 is a map of equal-pressure contours for a supine subject; the smaller the enclosed contour, the higher and more localized the pressure. Note the high-pressure regions under the head, shoulder blades, buttocks, thighs, calves, and heels; these are the sites most prone to pressure-induced injury.

According to Pearce (1986), it takes only 1 h to initiate tissue breakdown with local ischemia which produces tissue anoxia. The longer the period of tissue anoxia, the greater the tissue damage. With pressure-induced anoxia, the damage is usually not apparent immediately, although some skin blanching may be seen when the site is examined carefully. It usually takes many hours to days before the tissue damage has fully matured.

Factors that can exacerbate the development of pressure sores are age and disease in which the skin circulation is reduced. Drugs that produce vasoconstriction reduce skin circulation. Cross-clamping the aorta, as is performed during cardiopulmonary bypass, and the use of a tourniquet to obtain a bloodless field, compromise tissue capillary blood flow and predispose to tissue damage. Despite the fact that surgical patients are supported by foam pads to minimize areas of high contact pressure, some surgical procedures last many hours, during which time the patient is in the same position, which favors the genesis of tissue ischemia and pressure sores.

An interesting commentary on pressure sores was presented by Gendron (1980), who stated:

> No device on the market claims to be a complete substitute for routine relief of pressure. If routine turning of all patients is required every 2 h, and they rest on 7" thick hospital mattresses, it's obvious the standard 1½" foam pads on a steel table offer no real protection against pressure sores. The author observed the exact detailed outline of a table top machine screw head on a patient's side after a 3½ h procedure even though a 1½" pad was between the patient and the screw.

Pressure Sores

In a 100-patient study involving surgical patients ranging in age from 10 days to 81 years (mean age 39.11), Hicks (1970) reported that:

> The highest incidence of sores was in patients between 70 and 79 years of age, in patients whose general condition was poor, and in those on the operating table 4 h or longer. Every pressure sore occurred in an area associated with pressure experienced on the operating table.

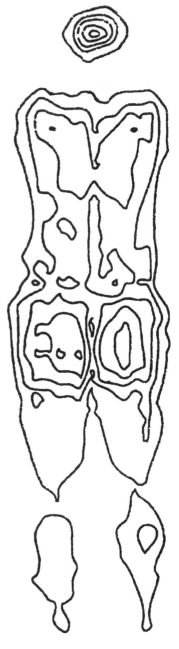

FIGURE 1 Isopressure contour map of a supine adult subject lying on a sleep surface. Higher pressures are under the head, shoulders, sacrum, thighs, calves and heels — the regions that support the body. (From Geddes, LA. Handbook of Electrical Hazards and Accidents. CRC Press, Boca Raton FL. 1995 By Permission.)

The importance of ischemic time was emphasized by Gendron (1980), who concluded that operative times of 2 h or less were not likely to result in pressure necrosis, while procedures lasting longer than 3 h predisposed the patient to skin injury from pressure.

Regarding the incidence and nature of pressure sores, *Health Devices* (1980) reported:

An often unrecognized source of skin destruction in the OR is prolonged immobility and pressure, which can lead to pressure necrosis. These injuries may resemble those caused by an ESU or hyperthermia unit — in fact, many lesions were originally suspected of having been caused by these devices. Most such injuries result from prolonged immobility, in which tissue pressure exceeds the critical closing pressure of subcutaneous blood vessels, so tissue ischemia exceeds physiologic tolerance. (ESU = electrosurgical unit)

Two cases of misdiagnosed thermal injury were reported by Chino and Nagel (1968), who stated:

A 63-year-old white man weighing 187 pounds was admitted with the diagnosis of bilateral iliac artery occlusion, arteriosclerotic heart disease, and diabetes mellitus. A warming blanket was placed on the operating room table, under the patient's hips and lower back, because of the anticipated prolonged surgical time. This blanket was covered by a double layer of drape sheet and the blanket's temperature regulator was set at 100° F. The patient underwent an aorto-bifemoral bypass with dacron graft placement and uneventful general anesthesia. The total time for the procedure was 6 h and 15 minutes. After several hours in the recovery area, the patient was returned to the operating room for further surgery. This procedure required an additional 1 h and 45 minutes. The postoperative course was then uncomplicated until the second postoperative day when the patient began to complain of severe discomfort in the sacral area. On examination he was found to have an area of burn over the sacrum estimated to be 40 percent third-degree, 60 percent second-degree, with strips of second degree burn extending over the buttocks. The area of burn corresponded to the location of the warming blanket used during surgery and the pattern of burn to the fluid channels in the coils of the warming blanket.

The second case was described as follows:

A 67-year-old white woman weighing about 150 pounds was admitted with gangrene of the right great toe and diabetes mellitus. After attempts to control the diabetes, she underwent an aortofemoral bypass graft under general anesthesia. A warming blanket covered by a sheet was placed under the patient's shoulders and mid back. The total operating time was 7 h and 15 minutes. On the second postoperative day the patient complained of "soreness" over her upper back. Examination revealed several areas of second-degree burn in a symmetrical pattern over the midthoracic area. Linear areas of erythema extended along the back and corresponded in spacing to the fluid channels in the warming blanket.

The authors believed that the injuries were due to the thermal blanket because the injury pattern corresponded to the channels in the blanket. However, temperature checking of the blanket revealed that there was not a significant temperature error relative to the thermostat setting. The temperature used was 100° F (37.8°C), which is well below the temperature for a first-degree burn, which is 45°C (Moritz and Henriques, 1947).

In view of the foregoing, it is necessary to seek another explanation for the injuries. Note that the duration of the operation for the first patient was 6 h and 15 min, plus 1 h and 45 min, i.e., a total of 8 h. For the second patient, the duration of the operation was 7 h and 15 min. Moreover, both patients were elderly and both had diseases that compromise the skin circulation. In view of all of these factors, these injuries must have been pressure sores.

Hair Loss Due to Pressure Necrosis

Remarkably clear examples of contact pressure necrosis, which produced hair loss, were given by Lawson et al. (1976), who reported the incidence of postoperative occipital alopecia (loss of hair on the back of the head). He stated:

> Postoperative alopecia is a minor complication of surgery, but a cosmetic disaster to the patient. Over a 3-year period, 60 cases of occipital alopecia were discovered in patients following open-heart surgery and 5 cases on other surgical services. In contrast to previous reports, 20 patients had alopecia one year later, presumed to be permanent. Extensive operations, with prolonged recovery and elective overnight mechanical ventilation, were common to all. Retrospective analysis and prospective studies clearly demonstrated that localized scalp pressure was the cause of the alopecia and that the duration of pressure determined the extent of the damage. Moving the patient's head at regular intervals during operation and recovery eliminated the alopecia. The type of head rest used did not modify the development of alopecia. Electrical injury and the use of heparin, hypothermia, electrocautery, or hypotension were eliminated as possible causes. Conclusive evidence correlating perioperative events with the formation of pressure sores in man has not been previously reported.

The foregoing cases demonstrate that tissue damage occurs at a site where tissue perfusion is compromised at a support point. It follows, therefore, that one should expect pressure-induced necrosis in the scapular, sacral, calf, and heel regions as predicted by pressure maps of supine subjects (see Figure 1 and Babbs et al., 1990). There are few data on prone and side-lying subjects, but the foregoing should alert one to identify the high-pressure points. Analysis of a large number of skin injuries can be found in a book by Gendron (1988). Thermal skin lesions due to electrosurgical grounding pads will be at different sites because such pads are not placed over bony prominences.

CHEMICAL INJURY

Introduction

When considering tissue injury due to chemical compounds, it is necessary to distinguish two types of response: (1) true chemical injury and (2) allergic response.

With the former, it is the nature of the chemical compound that produces the injury and with the latter, the host exhibits hypersensitivity to a substance (allergen); the response is typically unexpected and vigorous to the presence of very little allergen, which may be a very ordinary environmental substance. The correct term for the second type of response when it occurs on the skin is allergic contact dermatitis; all too often the term allergic is dropped. An allergic response is due to a prior exposure to a substance that endows the subject with an acquired hypersensitivity. Allergic responses will be described later in this chapter.

CHEMICAL TOXICITY

Valuable information about the effects of chemicals can be found in the Materials Safety Data Sheets (MSDS), the Drug Insert, and the Physician's Desk Reference (PDR); the contents of these sources are described in the chapter on product liability. The Occupational Safety and Health Administration (OSHA) requires that all personnel who handle chemical substances must have a copy of the MSDS and read it. Briefly, the MSDS identifies the name of the compound, its composition, brand name, physical and chemical properties, fire, explosion, and health hazard, first aid, antidote, and storage and disposal of the substance. The Drug Insert and the PDR identify indications, contraindications, dose, side effects, toxicity, and antidotes. The availability of such information often allows evaluation of the forseeability of an accident.

ETHYLENE OXIDE STERILIZATION

Ethylene oxide (ETO), which is a gas at atmospheric pressure and completely soluble in water, has been used as a sterilant since the early 1960s. Its value lies in the fact that the item to be sterilized can be placed in a sealed thermoplastic container which is then placed in the ETO sterilizing chamber. The first step in the process involves evacuating and warming the sterilizing chamber. Then ETO with a carrier gas (carbon dioxide or nitrogen) is admitted under controlled vacuum and humidity. The sealed container is bathed in the gas mixture for a prolonged period. Then the chamber is evacuated and the chamber (containing the item in the plastic container) is air washed several times with vacuum cycling to remove the ETO residue. This final step is necessary because ETO is a potent skin irritant (Sexton and Henson, 1950). There are standards that specify the maximum amount of ETO that can be present after sterilization. For example, the Health Industries Manufacturers Association (HIMA) and the New York Mt. Sinai Z-79 Committee have promulgated standards. There is an AAMI (1986) and an AAMI/ANSI standard (1988) that pertain to this issue.

A wide variety of medical items are sterilized with ETO. For example, all items that cannot withstand the heat of steam sterilization are candidates. In fact, it was development of the ETO sterilizer that gave birth to the disposable medical products industry. Familiar examples of items sterilized by ETO are medical instruments, hospital bedding, drapes, gowns, sheets, catheters, catheter electrodes, anesthesia equipment, etc.

Accidents with ETO-Sterilized Items

The following accidents occurred in the early days of ETO sterilization when residue controls were not so strict. However, the cases are presented to illustrate the kinds of mishaps that can occur when ETO residue is present.

Randell-Baker and Roberts (1969) called attention to the numerous reports of tissue reactions to plastics and rubber items after ETO sterilization. They stated:

> Reactions have included hemolysis, either in pump oxygenators or blood adminis-
> tration sets, burns to surgeons' hands from ETO-sterilized rubber gloves, tracheal
> inflammation and necrosis during prolonged intubation or tracheostomy, and possible
> thrombophlebitis following the use of intravenous tubing. Toxic stabilizers leaching
> out of polyvinyl chloride (PVC) plastics may be one cause of tissue reaction.

No references were cited for these responses, but Randall-Baker and Roberts made the following recommendations to avoid such difficulties:

> (a) adequate aeration of gas-sterilized materials for a minimum of five to seven days
> at 50 C for 6 to 8 h in a properly designed aerator with bacterial filters; (b) avoidance
> of the use of 3-ml polythene wrap plastics containing acid phthallic ester plasticizers
> which absorb ETO selectively, and any previously gamma-ray-sterilized items; (c)
> increased use of disposable items.

White (1970), who was then chairman of the ASA Subcommittee on Standardization, was concerned about the need to provide a sterile tracheal tube and anesthesia breathing circuit for each patient. He made the following seven recommendations:

1. Polyvinylchloride or rubber materials sterilized with ethylene oxide should not be used within SEVEN DAYS following sterilization, if stored at room temperature.
2. A properly designed aerator heated to 50 C may be used to reduce safe aeration time to 12 to 18 h.
3. Polyethylene (3 to 5 mil) and paper wrap are the best packaging materials. Nylon and polyvinilidine chloride (e.g., Saran Wrap) are less permeable to ethylene oxide; polyvinylchloride delays elution.
4. Polyvinylchloride objects which have been gamma-irradiated should not be resterilized with ethylene oxide because significant amounts of ethyl-enechlorohydrin will be formed.
5. Disposable items should be discarded after use because the by-products of later ethylene oxide sterilization may be injurious, because of ethylene chlorohydrin in particular.
6. Water droplets should be removed from material to be sterilized in order to prevent the formation of ethylene glycol.
7. Biological indicators should be used as a frequent check on the effectiveness of sterilization.

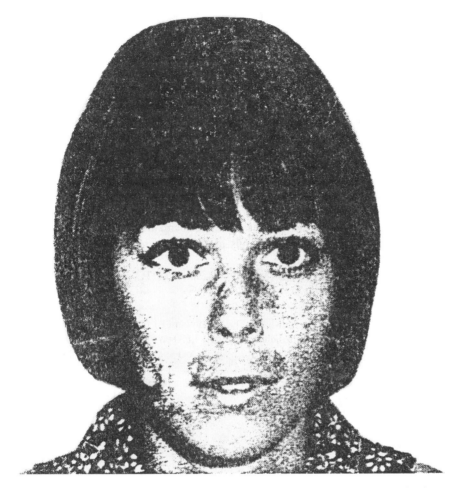

FIGURE 2   Facial injury due to a facemask sterilized with ETO. (From LaDage, L.H. *Plastic Reconstr. Surg.* 1970, 45(2): 179 By Permission.)

LaDage (1970) reported a case of facial skin irritation due to a face mask that had been sterilized with ETO. He stated:

The patient is a 21-year-old lady who underwent lengthy surgery under general anesthesia, which was administered with a mask. Apparently, the mask had been sterilized with ethylene oxide gas. She incurred severe burns of the facio-labial areas and on each side of her nose. What pressure and moisture had to do in aggravating the toxicity to produce this severity, I do not know.

Figure 2 is a photograph of the skin irritation reported by LaDage. An Editor's Note in his paper stated:

In some reports on this subject it would appear that the gas may be absorbed on the surface of impermeable materials (such as metals and glass) for a short time, but is actually absorbed into such permeable materials as rubber and some plastics (particularly, polyvinyl chloride). In the latter, it is said that forced ventilation for long periods (or exposure to room air for days, weeks, or months) may be necessary before use is free from risk.

Nineteen cases of skin irritation due to ETO-sterilized reusable gowns were reported by Biro et al. (1970); they stated:

Nineteen hospitalized women postoperatively suffered from severe burns of the buttocks and back from contact with reusable surgical gowns and drapes that had been sterilized with ethylene oxide and had not been properly aerated.

The lesions were described as erythematous, edematous with bullae (blisters) 1 to 5 cm in diameter. The bullae ultimately ulcerated in some cases and healed with scarring and hyperpigmentation.

Tests were performed to determine the amount of ETO residue on the gowns; Biro et al. (1970) reported:

Testing samples of reusable gowns that had been worn by the patients showed that the amount of ethylene oxide residue varied from 3,600 ppm ethylene oxide to 10,800 ppm ethylene oxide. The safe level for ethylene oxide gas recommended by both Health Industries Association (HIA) and Z-79 Committee of New York Mt. Sinai Hospital is 200 ppm (maximum). The levels of residual ethylene oxide in the implicated gowns were thus determined to be 16 to 50 times the safe level for skin contact. (ppm = parts per million)

Summary

The foregoing cases indicate the need for removing residual ETO from the sterilized item; failure to do so can result in tissue damage. Removing ETO residue requires appreciable time; therefore, the turn-around time for ETO sterilization can be days.

GLUTARALDEHYDE STERILIZATION

Glutaraldehyde is a powerful, water-soluble, biocidal agent that kills most microbial life, such as bacterial and fungal spores, tubercle bacilli, and viruses (Scott and Gorman, 1991). The biocidal action is enhanced by alkalization. Glutaraldehyde is available in concentrations up to 50%; however, a 2% solution is typically used to sterilize instruments and items that cannot withstand the heat of steam sterilization. Common preparations are Cidex, Glutarol, and Verucasep.

The device to be sterilized is first cleaned of debris and washed. It is then soaked in the glutaraldehyde solution. The biocidal efficacy depends on the concentration of the glutaraldehyde, the pH, the temperature, and the duration of soaking. It is advisable to use a nonmetallic container when sterilizing metallic devices, such as endoscopes, to avoid corrosion due to bimetallic contact because the glutaraldehyde solution can conduct electric current. Manufacturers of surgical instruments provide concentration and time recommendations for sterilization.

As with other chemical sterilizants, after the exposure phase, it is necessary to remove the glutaraldehyde residue adhering to the device. Soaking and repeated washing with sterile saline solution or sterile water removes the residue. Drying (if used) must occur in a germ-free environment.

Various authors have recommended different soaking times for sterilization. Corson et al. (1979) recommended that for routine laparoscope use between cases, a 15-min soak in Cidex is adequate, followed by a rinse in sterile water. A longer soak time (10 h) is necessary following use of an instrument in a patient with suspected infection. Shyu et al. (1992) recommended that transesophageal echocardiograph probes should be soaked in a gluaraldehyde solution for at least 20 min. Scott and Gorman (1991) reviewed the literature and recommend a 30-min immersion following use of an endoscope on a patient or carrier of hepatitis B or AIDS, and a 1-h immersion following use in tuberculosis patients.

Scott and Gorman (1991) stated:

> More recently, the interim report of the Working Party of the British Society of Gastroenterology recommended glutaraldehyde as a firstline disinfectant and proposed a 4-min soak as sufficient for inactivation of vegetative bacteria and viruses, including HIV and HBV. Many additional references have been made to the use of glutaraldehyde for rapid and safe disinfection of gastrointestinal endoscopy equipment.

Toxicity

The use of glutaraldehyde for chemical sterilization is now widespread and brings with it possible risks of toxic reactions to the individual handling the equipment during the sterilizing process and to the patient exposed to equipment treated with glutaraldehyde. In some cases this may bring a device in contact with the bloodstream.

The Materials Safety Data Sheet (MSDS) identifies the hazards of handling glutaraldehyde. For example, its vapors are irritating to the eyes; therefore, goggles or an eye shield should be worn. Vapor from a glutaraldehyde solution, if breathed, is irritating and will cause stinging sensations in the nose and throat, coughing, chest discomfort and tightness, breathing difficulty, and headache. Brief skin contact may cause mild to moderate local redness and possibly swelling. Prolonged contact may result in severe inflammation. Therefore, protective impermeable gloves should be worn.

Accidents with Glutaraldehyde Sterilization

Glutaraldehyde sterilization is now a mature procedure and there are few patient-related incidents. Numerous studies have been carried out on the microorganism level remaining on instruments and devices sterilized with glutaraldehyde preparations. Also, the absorption and rate of elution of glutaraldehyde from rubber and plastic goods have been documented. These issues were reviewed by Scott and Gorman (1991).

There have been a few incidents resulting from exposure to glutaraldehyde sterilizing solutions, which are typically 2% in strength. Using the results of a questionnaire, Axon et al. (1981) analyzed the responses from 52 centers in the U.K., each of which conducted about 500 endoscopic examinations annually. The analyses showed that 37% of the endoscopic units using glutaraldehyde solution as a disinfectant reported health problems among their staff, attributable to glutaraldehyde use. Axon et al. stated:

> 16 (37%) of those centers using glutaraldehyde had experienced problems with staff becoming sensitive to the disinfecting agent. A further questionnaire was sent to these centers and replies were received from all 16. These showed that 36 individuals had complained of 46 symptom complexes thought attributable to glutaraldehyde sensitivity. In 32, dermatitis had developed; these included 12 with symptoms in skin remote from the hands in addition to local dermatitis. 8 complained of conjunctivitis, and in 6 nasal irritation developed; 4 described this as sinusitis. (Information on allergic testing was not provided.)

Corrado et al. (1986) used provocative testing to determine allergic reactions in nurses who reported respiratory symptoms that they attributed to exposure to glutaraldehyde. Two of the four patients investigated had a confirmed reaction to glutaraldehyde.

ANTISEPTIC SOLUTIONS

In the late 1800s, Lister, a surgeon in Scotland, found that cleansing the skin with carbolic acid solution eliminated the infection associated with surgery. Then surgeons began to soak their hands in dilute carbolic acid to prevent bringing infectious agents into the surgical site. The use of rubber gloves arose from hand soaking in dilute carbolic acid. According to Haagensen and Lloyd (1946), it was Charles Goodyear, in collaboration with William Halstead, a surgeon at the Johns Hopkins Hospital, who introduced the use of rubber gloves to surgery in 1889. It is reported that Halstead's nurse developed lesions on her hands from carbolic-acid soaking. Halstead sought the aid of Goodyear to create rubber gloves, which were fabricated for the nurse. Others began to wear rubber gloves, which are now an essential component in asepsis.

Skin Preparation

Preoperative skin preparation is not a standardized procedure and uses many different antiseptic agents. Prior to the application of such agents, the skin may be washed with soap, shaved, or the hair removed by clipping or by the use of a depilatory. These pretreatments may affect the susceptibility of the skin to infection (Craig, 1986). However, irrespective of which antiseptic agent is used, it is essential to avoid its pooling because many of such agents can injure the skin if the pooling period is prolonged. Referring to skin injuries due to skin-preparation solutions, *Health Devices* (1980) reported:

Preventing chemical injury to the skin requires care on the part of the surgeon and the operating room staff. All prepping agents should be applied with great care and should not be allowed to pool beneath the patient or beneath a tourniquet.

A similar recommendation appeared in the FDA Drug Bulletin (1985) referring to an iodine tincture and stated:

The warning section of the labeling states that Hibitane Tincture must not be allowed to pool around the patient. Before the surgical procedure and electrocauterization are begun, the skin must be completely dry. Excess liquid should be removed with a sterile towel.

Iodine Compounds

Tincture of iodine, i.e., iodine in ethyl alcohol, supplanted carbolic acid as an antiseptic skin preparation and was used for some time until more recently, being supplanted by iodophors, i.e., organic substance-containing iodine. Several manufacturers provide such compounds under different trade names.

The toxicity of tincture of iodine and the iodophors is very low. Nonetheless, accidents have been reported. Llorens (1972) described two cases of skin injury due to povidone-iodine (Betadine). In cancer patients he described the first case as follows:

The night prior to the operation, the patient's abdomen was scrubbed with povidone-iodine, and again at the time of operation a 10-minute scrub with the same agent was done. A vaginal preparation with the same agent was also done. The surgical skin cleanser was used initially for approximately 10 minutes, followed by application of the povidone-iodine solution which was painted on with a gauze sponge. The patient had been previously placed on a water-circulating heating mattress. The surgical procedure lasted 4 h and 30 minutes. On the day following the operation, a reddened area over the sacrum was noted. This area became darkened, and eventually the superficial layer of epidermis desquamated.

Regarding the second patient, Llorens reported:

This patient had the same preparation as the previous patient, and a water-circulating heating mattress was also used. On the second postoperative day, a darkened area was noted over the lower back and sacral area. This measured approximately 20 by 20 cm, and was quite painful to the touch. As in the previous patient, this area also desquamated and with conservative measures healed spontaneously. She, too, was discharged on the fourteenth postoperative day.

A later statement in Llorens' paper offers a possible explanation for the injury. He stated, "Steps have been taken to prevent seepage of the scrub solution under the patient and in subsequent operations of this type, no further difficulty has been encountered."

Referring to the PDR, the following is stated for this antiseptic (Betadine): "Prolonged exposure to unabsorbed wet solutions may cause irritation." The fact that sacral contact pressure was probably high and heat was used may likely have exacerbated the injury reported by Llorens.

Feldtman et al. (1979) reported skin irritation due to Betadine; they stated:

We have noted 11 patients who have had their surgical wounds covered with a dressing containing 10% povidone iodine (Betadine). The wounds showed cutaneous erythema, induration, and also papulation, which conformed to the configuration of the dressing. All 11 patients who demonstrated this also showed a similar reaction to a 2 × 2 cm cotton pledget saturated with 10% povidone iodine. Diagnosis on ten of the 11 patients was suspect for altered immune state.

Note that the skin was exposed to liquid Betadine on a pledget which simulates pooling, a situation to be avoided according to the manufacturer. Later in the paper, the authors stated that they did not test for an immune response.

Another report recommending that wet iodine solutions should not be covered was presented by Howes et al. (1979), who stated:

Clinically, it is well known that solutions of iodine applied to the skin should not be covered with an occlusive dressing, a view supported by Dr. Morgan-Hughes's observations that erythema occurred in all areas painted with tincture of iodine and covered by Sleek (an occlusive dressing).

Another similar incident was reported by Duffy (1981), who stated:

After successfully cannulating the epidural space in a pregnant patient the anesthetic registrar covered the site with a gauze swab soaked in Betadine Antiseptic Solution (povidone iodine), as was his usual habit. At the suggestion of the assisting midwife this swab was then sprayed with a proprietary plastic skin and the whole area covered with a waterproof dressing.

At the opposite end of the spectrum of using an iodophor for wound-infection control is a report by Glick et al. (1985), who stated:

Continuous povidone-iodine irrigation is frequently used to treat mediastinitis after median sternotomy and has been considered safe and effective. We describe a 34-month-old patient with mediastinitis after median sternotomy who was treated with continuous povidone-iodine irrigation and who absorbed toxic quantities of iodine (total serum iodine, 9,375 µg/dl; normal range, 4.5 to 9.0 µg/dl). An unexplained metabolic acidosis developed, along with changes in mental status, and the patient died.

They concluded by stating:

Based on our clinical experience, experimental investigation, and critical review of the available literature, we believe that the routine use of povidone-iodine mediastinal irrigation is contraindicated. Whenever possible, antimicrobial irrigants should be picked based on specific bacterial sensitivities from cultures obtained at the time the irrigation tubes are placed. If this is not possible, or if microbial resistance occurs, then a highly dilute solution (1:1000) of povidone-iodine should be used. Administration of a highly dilute solution reduces the steady-state serum iodine concentration but not the antiseptic efficacy of povidone-iodine. In addition, if povidone-iodine is used, frequent serum iodine levels should be obtained to prevent excessive accumulation of iodine.

Response to Glick's paper by Rothwell (1980), on behalf of the manufacturer of Betadine, stated that the cause of the child's death was not established. Rothwell stated:

In my view, this isolated case report should not be extrapolated in absolute terms as stated in the article. Other prominent cardiovascular surgeons have found povidone-iodine to be highly effective when used preoperatively to prevent infection and postoperatively when infections have occurred as a result of operation. The intent of this letter is to bring some balance to the article by presenting reports in which povidone-iodine was used successfully when administered at appropriate dosage.

Mercury Compounds

Hodgkinson et al. (1978) commented on the effect of a mercury-containing antiseptic (thimerosal) and the exacerbating effect of pressure; they stated:

If the thimerosal has not been allowed to dry and has been trapped under the body of the patient in a pooled dependent position, like the buttocks for a patient in the stirrups, or under a tourniquet, the solvent may irritate the skin and result in a skin burn. Freon and alcohol as well as thimerosal usually evaporate after application. If these agents do not evaporate on contact with the skin and are trapped under a tourniquet or the buttocks of the patient or under drapes or dressings, they may irritate the skin. This irritation, coupled with pressure, leads to a situation analogous to that seen in the development of an acute accelerated decubitus ulcer: irritation, maceration, and pressure compounding each other to result in a skin burn or superficial ulcer in the skin. Friction from the underlying sheets has a variable role, as may the underlying heating blankets on the operating table.

ALLERGIC RESPONSES

An allergic response reflects a hypersensitive state acquired through prior exposure to a particular substance (allergen) and re-exposure produces an enhanced capability of the immune system to react. An allergen is any substance capable of producing a specific type of susceptibility. One may view an allergic response as an exaggeration of the body's defensive mechanisms. The allergic response may result from simple skin contact or inhalation, injection, ingestion, or implantation of a substance.

TABLE 1
Terms Used to Describe Allergic Skin Lesions

Term	Brief Definition
Bulla	Blister
Cyst	Fluid-filled sac
Dermatitis	Skin inflammation
Dermatographia	A condition in which tracing on the skin produces an elevated reddened track
Ecchymosis	Blood seen under the skin due to capillary damage
Eczema	Skin inflammation with vesication
Edema	Fluid accumulation in intercellular spaces
Erythema	Skin reddening
Induration	Hardening
Papule	Solid, skin elevation
Petechiae	Small round, purplish-red spots
Pruritis	Intense itching of the skin
Purpura	Purple
Stigmata	A spot or mark on the skin
Ulceration	Tissue disintegration and necrosis
Urticaria	Itchy, smooth, elevated skin patches of a different color
Vesicle	Small, fluid-filled sac
Wheal	Discolored, smooth, elevated skin region

The response can be in the respiratory, gastrointestinal, or nervous system, but cutaneous responses are perhaps the most frequently encountered allergic reactions. The respiratory responses are rhinitis and bronchial asthma. Among the gastrointestinal responses are vomiting, abdominal pain, and edema of the mouth, lips, and esophagus. Nervous-system responses include persistent headache, vomiting, and disturbances in the autonomic nervous system. A bewildering array of terms is used to describe allergic skin lesions; Table 1 presents a list of the terms along with simplified definitions.

Two interesting aspects of an allergic response are its unpredictability and recurrence in response to the allergen, despite a long dormant period when no allergen was present. The paragraphs that follow provide many examples of allergic response in association with the use of medical devices. The responses were not foreseen, nor could they be, unless (1) the subject knew of his/her allergy and (2) the material contacted contained the allergen. Although it is customary to inquire of allergies before administering drugs, the issue is usually not raised when using ordinary, frequently used, medical devices. However, the issue of forseeability of an allergic response can always be raised.

ALLERGIC CONTACT DERMATITIS

The prevalence of allergic contact dermatitis varies widely because its incidence is related to previous allergen exposure. Patch testing is used to identify persons suspected of being allergic to a substance. According to Larsen and Maibach (1992), surveys of normal subjects have shown that in a group of 1200 patch tests, sensitivity to the following was revealed: nickel 5.8%, neomycin 1.1%, ethylenediamine 0.43%, and benzocaine 0.17%. Among the common metallic sensitizers are nickel and chromium; some women cannot wear jewelry containing these elements. Larsen and Maibach tabulated many allergens; among the common items are benzocaine, black rubber, epoxy resin, formaldehyde, lanolin-alcohol, tetracycline, and thimerosal (a mercury-containing antiseptic).

The Patch Test

The patch test is used to identify an allergen. Although the techniques used in patch testing vary widely, the following is a simplified version. The test substance is applied to a piece of cloth or soft paper that is placed on intact skin and covered with an impermeable substance which acts as a backing and is affixed to the skin with tape. Often different concentrations of test substance are used to identify any threshold effect. After 48 h the patches are removed and the condition of the underlying skin is examined. A rash is evidence of a positive test. It must be recognized that the test is applied with each component of a substance that was suspected of producing an allergic response. The test can be designed to reveal the threshold concentration of the allergen.

Alcohol Allergy

Ethyl and isopropyl alcohols are used widely to disinfect the skin prior to its puncture by a needle. These alcohols are also used as a preservative in some skin preparations, as well as in electrode pastes to inhibit bacterial growth. Other compounds are added to prolong shelf life and there is remarkably little adverse reaction to these compounds. However, a small number of subjects are allergic to such preparations.

Two cases of allergic response to ethyl (potable) alcohol were reported by Drevets and Seebohm (1961) as follows:

A 67-year-old white widow was referred to the University Hospitals on Nov. 3, 1958, because of congestive heart failure. She had dyspnea on exertion, orthopnea, and progressively more distressing right upper quadrant abdominal pain intermittently for several months. She had noted itching and redness of the hands and fingers on the morning after drinking small amounts of alcoholic beverages the previous evening. She had first observed this 16 years previously. She drank alcoholic beverages, such as beer and wine, only on rare social occasions or for "medicinal" purposes. Because of the distressing symptoms following the ingestion of only two or three ounces, she had refrained from drinking alcoholic beverages during the previous year. There was no other history of clinical allergy.

Case 2 was:

A 25-year-old medical student, who lived in Hong Kong until he came to Iowa when 18 years old, was seen in the Allergy Clinic in January, 1960, with complaints of rhinorrhea and nasal stuffiness which he had had for 12 years. These symptoms had occurred during the period from mid August to early October for 7 years. He had not had eczema or asthma, but had experienced frequent respiratory infections during childhood. In addition to his respiratory complaints, he had noted a diffuse, erythematous, pruritic rash over his hands, wrists, elbows, and feet after drinking one to two ounces of one or another of several alcoholic beverages. This was first noted after the third or fourth time he ingested alcohol. Almost immediately after drinking, he had a diffuse erythema of the face which lasted for about 1 h. The rash appeared the next day and lasted 12 to 18 h. He rarely drank such beverages because of this reaction.

Patch tests were used to identify the allergens in these two cases; the authors reported:

In the study of the first patient, we applied patches with various dilutions of ethyl alcohol ranging from 5 to 70 percent. Two millimeter cubes of cotton soaked with the test solution and then squeezed free of excess fluid were put under the patches. These were applied to the arm or back for 24 h. Other tests with 70 percent methyl alcohol, 70 percent isopropyl alcohol, 35 percent butyl alcohol, 35 percent amyl alcohol, 50 percent acetone, 5 percent acetaldehyde, 5 percent formaldehyde, 1 percent formic acid, 1 percent phenol food coloring, and 1 percent glycerol were made. There were marked inflammatory reactions to the alcohols, but no response to the aldehydes, acetone, formic acid, glycerol, phenol, or food coloring. Patch tests with these same solutions caused no reaction on a control subject.

The patch test was followed by an interesting experiment described as follows:

We then gave the patient 60 ml of 90 proof whiskey through a nasogastric tube while she was fasting. In 30 minutes she began to appear giddy and in 2 h she complained of itching of the palms. Three hours later we noted minimal redness of the palms and backs of her hands. After 5 h, both surfaces of the patient's hands were moderately erythematous and pruritic. Eleven hours later intense pruritus developed over the arms, hands, anterior chest, neck, and thighs. These areas were markedly erythematous. Because of the intense pruritus and erythema of the skin, diphenhydramine hydrochloride and prednisone were given orally, and calamine with 1 percent phenol lotion was applied topically. These reactions were not as intense as those after the patch tests. At no time did she experience pain or any other systemic symptoms. The skin reaction gradually subsided. After 72 h there was no pruritus and only minimal erythema, which disappeared completely by the fifth day.

The response of the second patient was described as follows:

The second patient had a dermatitis to ingested alcoholic beverages, but the lesions could not be reproduced with topical application of alcohol.

The possibility that contaminants in ethanol could be responsible for dermatitis was considered by Fregert et al. (1965). They stated that:

The patient was a 62-year-old housewife; heredity — inquiry into her familial history revealed nothing of interest; previous illnesses — for 6 years she had had ulcerative colitis for which she had undergone gastroenterostomy; present illness — for the previous 12 years she had had a postthrombotic leg ulcer with periodic dermatitis. During an exacerbation of the dermatitis of the lower leg, epicutaneous tests were performed with the agents used for local treatment and routine test substances. The patient gave positive eczematous reactions to all test substances dissolved in ehanol. She also reacted positively to a patch test with ethanol.

After extensive patch testing, they concluded:

An eczematous contact dermatitis is described in a woman after application of low aliphatic primary alcohols, including methanol and ethanol. She reacted positively to ethanol but negatively to methanol. The corresponding acids gave negative reactions. Secondary and tertiary alcohols and ketones gave negative reactions.

Gas chromatography showed commercially available alcohols to contain contaminants, including aldehydes. However, even chromatographically pure ethanol produced dermatitis. Ethanol thus seems to possess allergenic properties in this patient but the possibility of a metabolite of ethanol, i.e., ethanal, being the allergen responsible cannot be excluded.

Fregert et al. (1969) pursued the allergic response to ethanol that was free of impurities. They summarized their results in four patients as follows:

Four female patients with eczematous reactions to lower aliphatic alcohols are described. One of them had skin symptoms also after consumption of alcohol and 3 had severe symptoms of the oral mucosa. Testing with gas-chromatographically pure methanol, ethanol, and 1-propanol showed positive reactions in all 4. They also reacted positively to unpurified 1-butanol. Of the secondary alcohols, 2 patients had reactions to 2-propanol and one to 2-butanol. None of the patients reacted to tertiary alcohol and only one patient reacted to croton aldehyde, which was one of the 5 aldehydes tested. All four reacted positively to patch test with beer and red wine.

Van Ketel and Tan-Lim (1975) described another case of allergy to ethyl alcohol; they reported:

A 52-year-old female patient was seen in a surgical ward after an operation for gallstones. Within 48 h after the operation an itching eruption developed on her abdomen underneath the gauze bandage which had been fixed with adhesive tape. The eruption had spread within 2 days beyond the bandage on the abdomen and thighs; rather ill-defined patches of erythema, papules, vesicles, and erosions were observed. It was diagnosed as contact eczema with an i.d. reaction. This patient was patch-tested also with Leukosilk (Beiersdorf), which showed no reaction. Patch tests with salts of iodine, chlorhexidene, ethanol 60% ketonated with oil of lavender, and non-ketonated ethanol 60% showed a strong positive allergic reaction after 48 h which proved that in this case an allergy to ethanol itself was present.

The cases just described demonstrate that some subjects are allergic to alcohols. As stated, alcohols are found in many substances that contact the skin and it follows that such subjects will exhibit an allergic response to alcohol-containing compounds.

Skin Rashes Associated with Recording Bioelectric Events

When bioelectric events, such as the electrocardiogram (ECG), electroencephalogram (EEG), electromyogram (EMG), electronystagmogram (ENG), etc., are recorded, an electrolytic preparation is placed between the metal electrode and the skin to make ohmic contact with the subject. Such preparations contain an electrolyte, usually sodium chloride, a gel, and a bacteriostatic agent. Sometimes the skin is first cleaned with alcohol; occasionally the skin is lightly abraded prior to placing the electrodes. In the early days of bioelectric recording, metal-plate electrodes were retained with rubber straps. Appearance of the self-adhering, disposable electrode has largely displaced the bare metal electrode for many applications. Nonetheless, in the disposable electrodes there is typically a metal electrode, a coupling gel containing the electrolyte, and a preservative; therefore, there exists the opportunity for one or more of these components to produce an allergic reaction in some subjects.

Electrocardiography (ECG)

Richardson et al. (1969) reported several cases of allergic contact dermatitis associated with routine electrocardiography; they stated:

> In a five-month period during 1969 and 1968, three individuals were seen at the University of Virginia Hospital with peculiar, discrete, rectangular areas of erythema and microvesiculation on the distal aspect of all four extremities. The areas of dermatitis in each patient corresponded to sites of electrocardiogram (ECG) electrode placement on the skin.
>
> Inquiry revealed that a prepackaged alcohol sponge had been utilized as a conductor between the patient's skin and the metal ECG electrodes. It was learned that it had become customary to substitute this same type of prepackaged alcohol sponge for electrode paste on the medical service.

A second observation of the nursing personnel was reported as follows:

> A few months later a nurse was seen who developed a hemorrhagic, vesiculobullous dermatitis on the tips of the fingers of the left hand, which cleared when she was on vacation and recurred when she returned to work. Upon questioning, it was learned that she frequently held the alcohol sponge in her left hand to cleanse a patient's arm prior to giving an injection with her right hand. Subsequently, another nurse with a similar history, who had an eczematoid eruption of her hands for many weeks, was brought to our attention. She had found that "alcohol sponges" were the cause of her eruption, and her dermatitis promptly cleared when she discontinued all contact with alcohol.

Patch tests were performed to confirm that the alcohol was the allergen. A similar case was reported by Schick (1981), who stated:

> ECG electrodes were placed using isopropyl alcohol swabs (Webcol Alcohol Prep, 70% alcohol, Kendall Co, Chicago) for conduction. Immediately following resuscitation, erythema in the areas of the ECG leads were noted on both arms and legs.

This progressed to blister formation and skin sloughing, followed by eschar development.

Para-chloro-meta-xylenol (PCMX) is an antibacterial agent that is used as a preservative in some electrode pastes. It is known that it is an allergen to some subjects, and Storrs (1975) reported several cases of allergic contact dermatitis caused by this agent. The first case was a young man who treated himself with several skin preparations some years earlier; Storrs reported:

> When he became an intern and surgery resident, he began to develop a vesicular eruption on several fingers of his right hand. He quite rightly suspected that Redux, electrocardiogram paste, was the culprit. When he was patch-tested to this paste, he developed a 3+ reaction within 12 h. Subsequently, he was tested to 0.5% PCMX in petrolatum and also had a 3+ reaction. He is now enlightened and his skin is clear as long as he avoids products which contain PCMX.

Storrs reported on other cases as follows:

> Two of our other patients also developed their dermatitis after exposure to Redux paste. Five patients were troubled by Carbolated Vaseline. One of these patients had trouble initially with Carbolated Vaseline and then developed dermatitis at the sites of the application of the electrodes with Redux paste when she received an electrocardiogram while hospitalized for treatment of her Carbolated Vaseline dermatitis.

In his paper, Storrs listed 35 familiar products that contain PCMX. Many of these products are widely used skin preparations, including vaseline.

Coskey (1977) reported a case of allergic contact dermatitis due to one component in an electrode paste used for recording the ECG. He stated:

> A 4-year-old boy was seen on March 23, 1976 because of persistent dermatitis on his chest and extremities. He had developed the eruption two months previously, shortly after an ECG had been taken. The eruption was confined to the areas where the electrode jelly had been used for contact between the skin and the electrodes.

Patch testing revealed that the subject was sensitive to tragacanth, a gum that was used as a binder in the electrode paste.

Over a 2-year period, Fisher (1977) encountered nine patients who developed allergic contact dermatitis associated with ECG recording. Five patients reacted to gels and/or pastes containing parabens, FD&C yellow #5, propylene glycol, PCMX, and pine oil. Two patients were allergic to the rubber straps that contained mercaptobenzothiazole. He described the reaction in these two patients as follows:

> Two patients were studied who acquired bandlike, erythematous, vesicular dermatitis at the sites of contact with the rubber straps used to fasten the ECG electrodes. Both patients showed a positive reaction to a piece of the rubber strap and to mercaptobenzothiazole. One patient gave a history of shoe dermatitis with previous hypersensitivity to mercaptobenzothiazole, which continues to be the most common cause of rubber sensitivity.

Fisher continued by reporting on a patient who acquired allergic contact dermatitis due to the nickel in the ECG electrodes; he stated:

> A twenty-six year old nurse at University Hospital acquired dermatitis at the sites where electrodes had been applied. It was at first suspected that she was allergic to the ECG pastes, but patch testing with the paste, which was performed elsewhere, gave negative results.
>
> The history revealed that she could not wear costume jewelry without acquiring dermatitis. A strongly positive patch test reaction to nickel sulfate was obtained, and the metal electrodes gave a strongly positive reaction to dimethylglyoxime, indicating the presence of "available" nickel in the metal electrode.

At that time, nickel-plated electrodes and German-silver electrodes were used for ECG. The latter alloy contains nickel, copper, and zinc, but no silver.

Fisher described his final case in which the patient was allergic to alcohol; he reported:

> A thirty-eight year old male had a sharp localized rectangular patch of vesicular dermatitis corresponding to the sites of the ECG cotton sponges which were used as conductors instead of ECG paste. This patient was found allergic, on patch testing, to the isopropyl alcohol used in the gauze pad and to ethyl alcohol. However, there was no systemic reaction from drinking alcoholic beverages.

Electroencephalography (EEG)

To record the EEG it is customary to adhere silver-disk electrodes to the scalp with collodion; alternatively, bentonite paste is used. Silver (1950) reported a case of allergic contact dermatitis when bentonite paste was used as the coupling agent; he reported:

> A 14-year-old white male with petit mal and grand mal attacks since 3 months of age was admitted for surgical consideration because of the focal nature of his attacks.
>
> Previous electroencephalograms had been made using collodion as the adhesive agent for scalp electrodes. Nine days following the use of Bentonite paste as the adhesive agent in electroencephalography, small annular, slightly elevated skin lesions were noted on the scalp; these had erythamatous centers and yellow borders.
>
> The site of the lesions corresponded to the points of application of the scalp electrodes. Patch testing proved that the patient was sensitive to Bentonite powder and not to the $CaCl_2$ or glycerin which comprise the paste.

Electronystagmography (ENG)

Nystagmus is a rapid movement of the eyeball which can be recorded by placing electrodes just lateral to the inner and outer canthis of the eye to obtain lateral eyeball movements. Electrodes can be placed supraorbitally and infraorbitally to record vertical motion of the eyeball. Such recordings are possible because there is a standing potential across the eyeball, the cornea being positive with respect to the back of the eyeball. For a discussion of recording methods, see Geddes and Baker (1989).

Strahan and Simmons (1968) reported two cases of skin lesions in an ENG study involving 600 patients. Placement of the electrodes was described as follows:

> The flat areas lateral to the lateral canthi are cleaned with an alcohol sponge and rubbed briskly with a wooden tongue blade after a standard electroencephalogram (EEG) electrode paste composed of bentonite, calcium chloride, and glycerin has been applied. The 9-mm silver electrodes are placed against the paste (not the skin) and secured with paper tape. A ground electrode is similarly placed on the forehead. In one of these patients (and in many others) a sodium chloride electrocardiogram ECG paste was used instead.

Strahan and Simmons described the two cases as follows:

> Case 1 — A 43-year-old psychiatrist had an electronystagmogram as part of a work-up for an unilateral sensorineural hearing loss. The patient and the technician who performed the test reported nothing unusual. Approximately four days later the patient noted raised, plaque-like red skin lesions bilaterally in the region of the electrode application. These lesions did not enlarge during the next week, however, several crusts were removed from their surfaces. By the third week the patient had bilateral, well circumscribed, erythematous bulky lesions which gradually calcified during the next two months. Since this time these lesions have diminished somewhat in size, but still remain as firm white blemishes.
>
> Case 2 — A 45-year-old housewife underwent electronystagmography as a part of a work-up for dizziness. The following day she noted a serous transudate from a flat but reddened 1-cm skin area in the region of electrode application on the left side. In the next two weeks this area crusted several times resulting in a raised erythematous plateau. By the end of three weeks, a hard, C-shaped white area appeared within the confines of this 1-cm raised erythematous lesion. This did not change in the next four weeks and surgical excision was performed for cosmetic reasons.

In analyzing their results, Strahan and Simmons ruled out electrical injury by testing their equipment and correctly pointing out that the skin lesions occurred in only 2 out of more than 600 patients. They concluded by stating:

> Though possible etiologies of these skin lesions include electrical burns, sensitivity to the electrode paste, and over-zealous preparation of the skin, the lesions were probably caused by a problem specifically related to the silver electrode and the individual's sensitivity.

Patch testing was not performed by Strahan and Simmons; therefore, the reason for the skin lesions is unknown. However, much earlier, Silver (1950) had reported allergic contact dermatitis due to benetonite paste.

ALLERGENIC METALS

Many of the commonly encountered metals and alloys produce allergic responses in some people. Among these metals are nickel, chromium, beryllium, mercury,

TABLE 2
Composition of Common Alloys

Alloy Name	Ingredients
Gold (14 kt)	Gold, copper, silver
Gold (white)	Gold, copper, nickel
Steel	Carbon, iron +
Stainless steel (316)	Manganese, carbon, phorphorus, sulfur, chromium, nickel, molybdenum
Monel	Copper, nickel
Sterling silver	Silver, copper +
German silver	Copper, zinc, nickel
Dental amalgam	Mercury, silver, tin, copper, zinc+
Brass	Copper, zinc
Vitallium	Chromium, molybdenum, iron, carbon, nickel, silicon manganese, cobalt

Note: + = plus other ingredients.

copper, gold, silver, and cobalt. Many people exhibit an allergic contact dermatitis when wearing items fabricated from these metals or their alloys. Of considerable importance are the allergic responses associated with implants made from these metals or alloys. Implants can be prosthetic devices, such as pins, plates, tooth fillings, dentures, and even bullets, shrapnel, or material deposited by tattooing. A few illustrative examples will be presented in the following paragraphs.

Table 2 lists a few of the commonly encountered alloys. An alloy is a uniform mixture of two or more metals, usually created by fusion, to obtain a material with desirable properties which are usually different from those of the components. Nonmetals are also used in alloys. Some believe that many pure metals are not allergens and it is the additives used to create the alloy that produce the allergic capability. For example, Gaul (1967) demonstrated this point by using controlled patch testing. Some of his patients had negative patch tests to pure gold, pure silver, and copper, but positive patch tests to nickel, 14-karat gold rings, and sterling silver rings. Although this may be true, it is surprising to note that an allergy can result from exposure to a single component in an alloy and this component can be a metallic element, as, for example, nickel in stainless steel.

There is some controversy about the allergic properties of the salt of a metal and the pure metal. For example, in a case reported by Comaish (1969), patch testing to metallic gold was negative, although 2% gold chloride produced a positive test reaction. From the foregoing examples, it appears that an allergic response can result from exposure to a pure metal, as well as its salt.

Nickel

Five cases of allergic contact dermatitis subsequent to earlobe piercing were reported by McKenzie (1967). All subjects were young ladies (16 to 20 years) who had their earlobes pierced to wear ornamental earrings. Sterling silver and 14-kt gold contacted the pierced sites and patch testing for nickel gave positive results in four of five subjects; the no-response in one case was not explained.

Because ladies will continue to have their ears pierced, Gaul provided the following recommendations:

> Ear lobes should be pierced by approved techniques. Channel patency should be maintained with gold or silver wires of known composition, or black silk thread. Earrings should not be worn until the channels are completely epithelized. The person piercing the ear should follow through with his subjects and direct them to a source of earrings which are known to be nonirritating and nonsensitizing.

Over a 12-month period, Watt and Baumann (1968) encountered 17 female patients who developed an allergic contact dermatitis to nickel as a result of earlobe piercing; they reported their cases as follows:

> The ages of our patients ranged from 15 to 23 years. The time interval between the earlobe piercing and the onset of a draining earlobe dermatitis was between two and four weeks. In one patient the reaction occurred many years after piercing, but shortly after the use of some "cheap" earrings. In approximately one half of the cases the dermatitis spread to involve other areas where metal was in contact with the skin. In two patients a generalized dermatitis of autoeczematization ensued.
>
> All 17 of the women developed strongly positive eczematous reactions to nickel patch tests.

To prevent such an occurrence, they recommended:

> A history of nickel allergy is an absolute contraindication to earlobe piercing procedures.

Barranco and Soloman (1972) reported a case of nickel dermatitis in a 20-year-old lady who had her ears pierced prior to a surgical implant; they reported:

> A 20-year-old white woman had her ears pierced in 1967. In July 1968, a Hauser procedure was done on the left knee for a chronically dislocated patella. A stainless steel screw was used to secure a transferred tendon in its new location. The patient experienced no difficulty with this procedure. The same procedure was done on the right knee in June 1969; again, a stainless steel screw was used to reattach the transferred tendon. This time the procedure was complicated by a wound dehiscence and secondary closure.

In October 1969:

> An extensive eruption on the chest and back developed. This was a subacute eczematous dermatitis involving the skin of the shoulders, midback, buttocks, abdomen and breast. She was treated with both topical and systemic corticosteroids with only minimal improvement. She then disappeared from follow-up until November 1970. At this time the dermatitis was noted to be widespread as before, but also in areas

of contact with jewelry such as the earlobes, neck, and ring fingers. It was thought that she had a contact dermatitis most likely to nickel.

Patch testing with nickel sulfate gave a 4+ result and Barranco continued:

Out of sheer desperation, the stainless steel screws were considered a possible cause of the dermatitis, and the orthopedic surgeon begrudgingly removed them. The day following removal of the screws, the erythema had markedly subsided with very little itching present. Seventy-two hours later, she was essentially clear of her dermatitis, with no itching. Her treatment continued to be only topical corticosteriods.

Five days following removal of the screws, closed patch testing was done with pure nickel, nickel sulfate, pieces of the stainless steel screw recently removed from the patient, and a current routine chemical patch-testing tray. All tests were negative except for a 4+ reaction to nickel, nickel sulfate, and the stainless steel screw.

Barranco continued:

The orthopedist still doubted that the stainless steel screw could be the cause of her dermatitis and reapplied the screw to the skin of the back. In a period of 4 h, generalized pruritus and erythema again developed.

A case of allergic contact dermatitis due to the nickel in a chromium–cobalt alloy in a partial dental plate was reported by Brendlinger and Tarsitario (1970), who stated:

A 25-year-old mother of three was first seen by a dermatologist on January 30, 1968. She had generalized pruritic eczematous eruptions on the trunk, arms, and legs. Treatment with topical corticosteriod preparations gave her some relief. She was released from treatment after one month.

On August 29, she returned with a dermatitis on her ring finger. Just before this time she began working for an electronics firm. It was thought that the dermatitis was due to the metal in her gold ring. In spite of repeated topical corticosteroid and hydration treatments the dermatitis became worse. By October she had eczematous dermatitis over her entire body. It was particularly severe wherever metal touched her skin: ear, fingers, wrist, waist, and so on. Her hands were becoming fissured and erythematous. Neither topical nor systemic corticosteroids helped.

Numerous laboratory tests were performed without resolving the problem. Treatment consisted of corticosteroids and avoidance of metal contact by wearing gloves. The report continued:

In November she began to complain of soreness in her mouth. She was referred to the oral surgery clinic where it was discovered that she was wearing an all-cast chrome cobalt-type removable partial denture to replace her maxillary right central incisor. This had not been observed or considered during her previous treatment. The mucosa under the metal was denuded of epithelium and she still had generalized eczematous lesions over most of her body. Although the probability was low, the possibility of sensitivity to the partial dentures was pursued. The patient was referred to the prosthodontic section of the dental clinic for further evaluation.

An all-acrylic resin treatment partial denture was made to replace the metal denture. The acrylic resin was heat cured for 12 h. A gold-fixed prosthesis was temporarily ruled out until more specific allergens could be identified. The day after the insertion of the acrylic resin denture the patient began to improve. The itching stopped and the skin lesions healed. All cortisone and antibiotics were stopped. Within three days she became completely clear of symptoms and signs.

The dermatology clinic confirmed the patient's sensitivity to chrome and nickel by skin testing pure samples of these metals provided by a manufacturer of a chrome-cobalt alloy and the metallurgy department of the University of Illinois. All chrome cobalt alloys contain enough nickel to produce allergic reactions in sensitive individuals.

Of her own volition, the patient inserted the metal partial denture one evening and by the next morning she began to break out with lesions again. She came into the oral surgery clinic that morning. After pictures were taken she removed the metal denture and reinserted the acrylic resin treatment denture. The next day she was clear of lesions.

McKenzie (1967) reported an allergic response to the implantation of a Vitallium nail used to repair a fracture of the neck of the femur, he stated:

On 11 January 1965 a woman of 65 sustained a fracture of the right femoral neck. The next day a Smith-Petersen Vitallium nail was inserted under halothane anesthesia. On the day after operation pruritus and generalized urticaria developed, and these symptoms persisted for the next 10 months. During this time there was radiological healing of her fracture, but there was little weight-bearing on the limb on account of anginal congestive cardiac failure and three episodes of cerebral thrombosis. A right-sided hemiplegia followed one of these strokes.

On 8 December she was admitted to the Norfolk and Norwich Hospital for investigation of urticaria. Her major physical findings were right-sided flaccid hemiplegia, generalized urticaria, and dermographism.

After considerable laboratory work, patch testing was performed which revealed:

An eczematous response to a solution of 2% nickel sulfate at 48 h. A similar response was produced by a Vitallium nail strapped to the thigh for 48 h. During patch testing there was no increase in severity of urticaria, but severe non-eczematous periorbital oedema developed at 48 h and resolved within the following 12 h. A scratch test with 2% nickel sulfate solution resulted in an itching wheal (3 cm) at 10 minutes, and was associated with patchy erythema and swelling of the same forearm for 1 h.

Since the patient was bedfast and her fracture had healed clinically, the nail was removed on 10 January 1966 under local anesthesia. Within 24 h spontaneous urticaria resolved but dermographism persisted. Exquisite and troublesome dermographism was still present one year after removal of the nail.

Note that Table 2 identifies the ingredients of Vitallium, one of which is nickel.

An interesting case of nickel allergy was described by Pegum (1974) in which the time between allergy identification and an allergic response was more than one quarter century. He stated:

> A 38-year-old woman had reacted to white metal since the age of 12. At the age of 35 an osteotomy of the left hip was performed and a Wainwright stainless-steel plate was inserted (nickel 8–12%, chromium 17–20%, manganese 2%, molybdenum 2.5–3.5%). All went well for some three years, and then dermatitis of various parts of the skin and sterile suppuration around the plate developed. The suppuration and the dermatitis resolved after the plate was removed. Patch tests to nickel and chrome, as well as to the central plate, were positive. It will be evident that not only did dermatitis develop in our patient, but also "rejection" of the implant."

Mercury

Mercury is found in the amalgam used to fill cavities in teeth. Foussereau and Laugier (1966) reviewed the literature on allergic responses to such dental fillings. From 1934 to 1951 four cases of allergy to the mercury in the amalgam were reported; the allergy was confirmed by patch testing.

Allergic responses to the deposition of mercury salts in tattoo procedures were reported by Foussereau and Laugier (1966). The red pigment is mercury sulfide, the blue is cobalt aluminate, and the green is chromium oxide. In addition to mercury, potassium bichromate was shown to be an allergen associated with tattoos.

Gold

Pure gold (24 kt) is a soft malleable element that is rarely used in this form. It is alloyed with a variety of elements such as copper and silver to harden it.

Forster and Dickey (1949) described an unusual case of gold allergy; they stated:

> On admission here, the visual acuity of the right eye was hand movements; of the left eye, no light perception. The diagnosis was bilaterial congenital dislocated lenses with uveitis and secondary glaucoma. The left eye was blind and painful. Enucleation was performed and a 14-karat gold ball, 14 mm in diameter, of the standard variety used at that time, was implanted into Tenon's capsule. Recovery was uneventful. A glass prosthetic shell was procured.

After a stormy time dealing with apparent infection, it was ultimately suspected that allergic contact dermatitis to gold may be present. It was determined that 14-k gold is composed of 60% fine gold, 35% copper, and 5% silver and tin. Standard, closed-patch tests were made with 1% copper sulfate, gold sodium thiosulfate, silver, copper, tin, and gold leaf, the 14-kt ball, and the plastic prosthetic eye. The gold salt, gold leaf, gold ball all gave 4+ responses.

The report concluded by stating:

> At the time of this report two years have elapsed since removal of the gold ball and the patient has had no recurrence of her disfiguring orbital discharge which for 3 years prior to removal of the gold ball had made her life miserable.

An unusual dental case was reported by Elgart and Higdon (1971), who summarized it as follows:

> Gold sensitivity (the eighth reported case, the seventh proved case) occurred in a 27-year-old woman. This is the first instance where a dental appliance was involved. The gingival mucosa sloughed following contact with a gold crown, and previous sites of contact dermatitis to jewelry flared.

Reporting on the case, Elgart stated:

> A 27-year-old woman had no allergic problems until 1967, when her ears were pierced. Following this, she developed an eczematous reaction to gold earrings, and had to stop wearing them. She then found that she could no longer wear her gold rings or wristwatch. In each instance, the reaction was characterized by an erythematous, scaly, and weeping dermatitis. It was noted to subside a few days after she stopped wearing the offending jewelry. The problem seemed more severe during the summer months.
>
> In October 1969, a gold crown was placed on a left lower bicuspid. Within a few days, there was irritation of the gingival mucosa around it, and an eczematous dermatitis again appeared under her ring. When she removed the ring, the erythema did not subside.
>
> The lesions were treated with ointment with little success. Extensive patch testing was performed with gold (auric) tricholoide, 0.5% aqueous. A positive response was noted within 24 h, with vesicles, severe erythema, and edema. Exacerbation of previous locations of her dermatitis again occurred.
>
> In July 1970, because of repeated episodes of difficulty with her gums and hand dermatitis, the gold crown was removed. Within a week, the oral lesions had improved, and at the end of a month, all traces of irritation of the gingival mucosa and of the hands disappeared.

Metals in Military Missiles

Metals can be implanted by bullets and shrapnel. Foussereau and Laugier (1966) reported that grenade and mortarshell cast iron and American shell steel contain nickel and chromium. They reported the interesting case of:

> Mr. O., aged 43, a former bricklayer, had been working as a chromium and nickel plater since 1960. In December 1960 an eczema broke out, for the first time, under his watch on his left wrist and was aggravated through his work. Metal allergy was proved by the strong positivity of the skin tests (+++ to chromium, nickel, and cobalt). The patient changed his occupation, becoming a warehouseman in a spinning factory. His condition remained satisfactory up to 1963, when a swelling occurred on his left forearm, becoming fistulas within a few weeks and accompanied by an outbreak of eczema on the upper limbs, particularly on the left side. As confirmed by X-ray, the fistula was due to a piece of grenade shrapnel which had embedded itself in the patient's left elbow in 1942. On March 14th, 1963, because of the fistulization and the metal allergy, the shrapnel was removed. Since then the eczema has ceased to develop in the form of acute episodes.

Allergic Response to Bed Linens

These days there are few allergic responses to bedlinens owing to the considerable improvements in hospital laundries and the reduced time patients remain in hospitals. Nonetheless, there is some concern that antibacterial and softener residues from the washing cycle are not totally removed by the rinse cycles. Parenthetically, washing is carried out at a highly alkaline pH and acid correction (souring) is used later to make the pH neutral (e.g., about 7.0).

A case of severe asthma and urticaria induced by an antibacterial agent (phenylmercuric proprionate, PMP), used in laundering bedclothes, was reported by Matthews and Pan (1969). The subject was described as follows:

> A thirty-four-year-old male resident physician was first seen on March 30, 1962, complaining chiefly of asthma and urticaria. His mother has asthma. As a child, in Europe, the patient had urticaria which occurred only after eating pork, green beans or strawberries. He had experienced reactions, probably of an allergic nature, to tetanus antitoxin, penicillin, erythromycin, and perhaps sulfaguanidine. After coming to this country (Cincinnati) in the summer of 1960, he had symptoms typical of allergic rhinitis. This difficulty subsided in late September but recurred the following June. He moved to Ann Arbor in July 1961. During the summer his rhinitis became progressively worse, and for the first time he experienced mild asthma. All symptoms promptly subsided on a trip to Europe in September with no recurrence of his rhinitis upon returning to Ann Arbor in October.
>
> During the fall of 1961, however, he began to have nocturnal attacks of asthma. These progressed in severity and occurred almost exclusively while in his bed in the Interns' and Residents' Quarters (night or day) and would subside within an hour or two after leaving his room. He was free of symptoms in his room if he did not lie on the bed. However, while assigned to the Tuberculosis Service in February 1962 he noticed that he would have asthma at work if he wore a gauze mask but no asthma if he wore a paper mask. At this time he also started to have urticaria and angioedema. These lesions usually broke out at night or in areas of contact with his white uniforms.

The report continues with a detailed account of subsequent attacks and describes the extensive testing that identified PMP as the allergen. The report concluded by stating:

> The patient was exceptional in giving a passively transferable immediate wheal and erythema skin test reaction to relatively low molecular weight compounds. Other immunologic studies were negative except for *in vitro* histamine release from leukocytes by the allergen. The patient also gave skin test reactions to other phenylmercuric compounds. In high concentrations these compounds are irritants. They are widely employed as antibacterial and antifungal agents in agriculture, industry, and medicinals, and are used in washing the linens of many hospitals.

Rycroft (1976) reported on 9 cases of dermatitis associated with sheets and pillow cases; he stated:

Since April 1975 we have seen nine patients with widespread dermatitis who had recently purchased cheap Canadian bed sheets. Three days to two weeks after starting to use the sheets they had developed severe itching and burning sensations, especially at night. When pillow cases had also been purchased, redness of the ears and puffy eyelids were early complaints. In some cases several members of one family were affected, and in others one bed partner was spared.

The report continued:

Patch tests with the patients' own sheets produced negative results in five out of eight cases tested, and there were no positive patch test results with formaldehyde. Only one patient reacted to a standard formaldehyde clothing resin patch test. Laundering the sheets helped in only one case, in which tolerance was reported after three washes. Once the patients stopped using the sheets the rash usually resolved in three to four weeks.

Curran (1988), a hospital laundry manager, recommended a procedure to minimize skin irritation from sheets. He stated:

In our operation, all of our wash persons sign a policy statement that they *Must* test each and every load of linen before they take it out of the washer. The test is simple and easy. Just put one drop of pH indicator on a piece of linen in that load, if it turns orange-red, the load is at a pH level of 5 or 6, the pH of normal skin. If it turns green, then you have alkali left in the linen. This could cause skin irritation. If this happens, the load of linen must be put back through the sour and softener cycle to insure the linen comes out at the proper pH level. (The term "sour" means acidification.)

ALLERGIC RESPONSE TO RUBBER AND PLASTICS

Rubber is known to be an allergen, as described in a preceding paragraph relating to the use of rubber bands to secure ECG electrodes to the extremities. According to Larsen and Maibach (1992) it is some of the additives, notably, mercaptobenzothiazole, tetramethyl-thiuram, and others, that endow rubber with its allergenic properties.

We live in a world in which we are surrounded by objects made of plastics or covered by plastic and the incidence of allergic reaction is small, but finite. For example, Mather et al. (1993), after encountering skin reactions due to nylon catheters in nine patients, sought to determine the incidence of such an event. They reported as follows:

After computer searches and direct inquires to 11 manufacturers, we can find no reports of any similar reaction to any epidural catheter.

The responses of the six patients who received epidural catheters were similar; one case will be presented as follows:

A healthy 66-year-old woman was admitted for total abdominal hysterectomy and bilateral salpingo-oophorectomy. She gave a history of allergy to rubber, horse serum, adhesive bandages, and several types of tapes.

Before induction of general anesthesia, an epidural catheter was inserted at the L3-L4 interspace and established using 2% lidocaine with epinephrine (2% w lidocaine). Following the Acute Pain Service protocol, 5% providone-iodine (Betadine) spray was used prior to catheter placement. Thereafter, tincture of benzoin and a Tegaderm dressing (10 × 30 cm) were used to secure and cover the catheter.

For postoperative analgesia she received an epidural dose of 2 mg morphine (1 h before the end of surgery) and was subsequently prescribed 2 mg epidural morphine every 6 h as needed. On the second morning after surgery (40 h after epidural catheter insertion) she complained of "soreness" only at the point of entry of the catheter, where there was also a "circle of inflammation and a small amount of swelling." It was decided that the best course of action would be to remove the catheter and extend the course of perioperative antibiotics (cephalexin). Upon removal there was a small amount of serous discharge, but it also became evident that there was an inflammatory "trail", which traced the exact course of the epidural catheter from her lower back, up to and over her shoulder. The "trail" was about 5 to 6 mm wide and persisted, albeit faded, until her discharge on postoperative day 6.

Clinically, each of the cutaneous reactions appeared identical. All six patients had a reddened, non-raised trail, which began at the site of catheter insertion and coursed along the back. Each trail appeared simultaneously and faded simultaneously over the length of catheter-skin contact. The observed time to onset ranged from 40 h to several days with resolution over 1 to 3 days. Additionally only case 4 had associated blistering; only cases 1 and 3 had palpable swelling at the site of catheter entry; and only cases 1 and 3 complained of localized itching. Clinically, the course and dimensions of the inflammatory "trails" in our patients corresponded exactly with the epidural catheters. However, other local factors may have caused this reaction.

They summarized by stating:

Since an allergic reaction to an epidural catheter has not been reported, it can be presumed to be a rare event. This makes the likelihood of six cases of allergy in a matter of weeks improbable. We, therefore, considered any other recent changes in our practice that might coincide with these occurrences. However, nothing has been changed in 6 yr. We are using the same antiseptic, catheters, dressings, and drugs. The manufacturer states that there have been no recent changes to the manufacturing process of their catheter.

CONCLUSION

Although allergic responses are quite uncommon, they require good detective work to identify the allergen. Fortunately, patch testing or disappearance of the allergic response when the allergen is removed is all that is required to identify the allergen.

REFERENCES

AAMI. Recommended Practice for Determining Residual Ethylene Oxide in Medical Devices. 1986. Association for the Advancement of Medical Instrumentation, 3330 Washington Blvd., Suite 400, Arlington, VA 22201-4598.

AAMI/ANSI. Guideline for Industrial Ethylene Oxide Sterilization of Medical Devices. 1988. Association for the Advancement of Medical Instrumentation, 3330 Washington Blvd., Suite 400, Arlington, VA 22201-4598.

Axon, A.T.R., Banks, J., Corket, R., et al. Disinfection in upper digestive tract endoscopy in Britain. *Lancet* 1981, May 16: 1093–1094.

Babbs, C.F., Bourland, J.D., Graber, G., et al. A pressure-sensitive mat for measuring contact pressure distribution of patients lying on hospital beds. *Med. Instr. Technol.* 1990, 24: 363–370.

Barranco, V.P. and Soloman, H. Eczematous dermatitis in nickel. *J.A.M.A.,* 1972, 110: 1244.

Biro, L., Fisher, A.A., and Price, E. Ethylene oxide burns. *Arch. Dermatol.* 1974, 110: 924–925.

Brendlinger, D.L. and Tarsitario, J.J. Generalized dermatitis due to sensitivity to a chrome cobalt removable partial denture. *J.A.D.A.* 1970, 81: 392–394.

Chino, M.J. and Nagel, E.L. Thermal burns caused by warming blankets in the operating room. *Anesthesiology* 1968, 29(1): 149–150.

Comaish, S. A case of contact hypersensitivity to metallic gold. *Arch. Derm.* 99: 720–1969.

Corrado, O.J., Osman, J., and Davies, R.J. Asthma and rhinitis after exposure to glutaraldehyde in endoscopy units. *Hum. Toxicol.* 1986, 5: 325–327.

Corson, S.L., Block, S., Mintz, C., et al. Sterilization of laparoscopes. *J. Reprod. Med.* 1979, 23: 49.

Corson, S.L., Dole, M., Kraus, R., et al. Studies in sterilization of the laparoscope. *J. Reprod. Med.* 1979, 23: 57.

Coskey, R.J. Contact dermatitis caused by electrode jelly. *Arch. Dermatol.* 1977, 113: 839–840.

Craig, C.P. Preparation of the skin for surgery. *Today's OR Nurse* 1986, 8(5): 17–21.

Curran, C.C. Laundry plays roll(e) in pressure sore prevention. *Health Care Systems* 1988, 25(a): September.

Drevets, C.C. and Seebohm, P.M. Dermatitis from alcohol. *J. Allergy* 1961, 32(4): 277–282.

Duffy, B.L. Betadine burn. *Anesth. Intensive Care* 1981, 9(4): Correspondence.

Elgart, M.L. and Higdon, R.S. Allergic contact dermatitis to gold. *Arch. Dermatol.* 1971, 103: 649–653.

Food & Drug Administration. FDA Drug Bull. (Washington, D.C.) 1985, 15(1): 9.

Feldtman, R.W., Andrassy, R.J., Page, C.D., et al., Providone-iodine skin-sensitivity observed with possibly altered immune status. *J.A.M.A.* 1979, February: 487.

Fisher, A.A. Dermatologic hazards of electrocardiography. *Cutis* 1977, 20: 686.

Fisher A.A. Safety of stainless steel in nickel sensitivity. *J.A.M.A.* 1972, 221: 1232.

Forster, H.W. and Dickey, R.F. A case of sensitivity to gold ball orbital implant. *Am. J. Ophthal.* 1949, 32: 659–662.

Foussereau, J. and Laugier, P. Allergic eczemas from metallic foreign bodies. *Trans. St. John's Hosp. Dermatol. Soc.* (London) 1966, 57: 220–225.

Fregert, S, Hakanson, R., Rossman, H., et al. Dermatitis from alcohols. *J. Allergy* 1965, 34: 404–408.

Fregert, S., Groth, O., Hjorth, N. et al. Alcohol dermatitis. *Acta. Derm. Venerol.* 1969, 49: 493–498.

Gaul, L.E. Development of allergic nickel dermatitis from earrings. *J.A.M.A.* 1967, 200: 186–188.

Geddes, L.A. and Baker, L.E. *Principles of Applied Biomedical Instrumentation.* 3rd ed. 1989. John Wiley & Sons, New York.

Gendron, F.C. *Unexplained Patient Burns.* 1988. Quest Publishing (now Lippincott-Raven Press), Brea, CA.

Gendron, F.G. "Burns" occurring during lengthy surgical procedures. *J. Clin. Eng.* January–March 1980, 5: 19–26.

Glick, P.L., Gugielmo, B.J., Tranbaugh, R.F., et al. Iodine toxicity in a patient treated by continuous providone-iodine mediastinal irrigation. *Ann. Thoracic Surg.* 1985, 39(5): 478–480.

Haagensen, C.D. and Lloyd, W.E.B. Anesthesia and antisepsis. In *New Worlds in Medicine.* Wood, H.B., Ed., 1946. R.M. McBride, New York.

Health Devices. Hazard: Skin injury in the OR and elsewhere. *Health Devices* 1980, 9(12): 312. Emergency Care Research Institute. 5200 Butler Pike, Plymouth Meeting, PA 19462-298

Hicks, D.J. An incidence of pressure sores following surgery. In *ANA Clinical Sessions* (1970). 1971. Appleton-Century-Crofts, 1971. New York.

HIMA. Guidelines for the Analysis of Ethylene Oxide Residues in Medical Devices. Document No. 1, Vol. 1. 1980. Health Industries Manufacturers Association, 1200 G St NW, STE 4000, Washington, D.C. 20005.

HIMA. Ethylene Oxide Residues on Sterilized Medical Devices. Report 88-6. 1988. Health Industry Manufacturers Association, 1200 G St NW, STE 4000, Washington, D.C. 20005.

HIMA. Sterilization in the 1990s. Report 89-1. 1989. Health Industry Manufacturers Association, 1200 G St NW, STE 4000, Washington, D.C. 20005.

Hodgkinson, D.J., Irons, G.B., and Williams, T.J. Chemical burns and skin preparation solutions. *Surg. Gynecol. Obst.* 1978, 147: 534–536.

Howes, J.G., Baud, C. and Kirwan, P. Iodine and acetone-containing plastic spray dressing. *Br. Med. J.* 1979, February: 487.

LaDage, L.G. Facial irritation from ethylene oxide sterilization of anesthesia mask? *Plastic Reconstructive Surg.* 1970, 45(3): 179.

Larsen, W.G. and Maibach, H.I. Allergic contact dermatitis. In *Dermatology.* 3rd ed. 1992. Moschella, S.L. and Hurley, H.J., Eds. W.B. Saunders, Philadelphia.

Lawson, N.W., Mills, N.L., and Ochser, J.L. Occipital alopecia following cardiopulmonary bypass. *J. Thor. Cardiovasc. Surg.* 1976, 71: 342–347.

Llorens, A.S. Reaction to providone-iodine surgical scrub associated with radical pelvic operations. *Am. J. Obst. Surg.* 1972, November 15: 834–835.

Mather, C.M.P., Anaes, F.C., and Neuman, M. Inflammatory cutaneous reactions to epidural catheters. Anesthesiology 1993, 78(1): 200–204.

Matthews, K.P. and Pan, P.M. Immediate type hypersensitivity to phenylmercuric compounds. *Am. J. Med.* 1968, 44: 310–318.

McKenzie, A.W. Urticaria after insertion of Smith-Peterson vitallium nail. *Br. Med. J.* 1967, 4: 36.

Moritz, A.R. and Henriques, F.C. The relative importance of time and surface temperature in the causation of skin burns. *Am. J. Pathol.* 1947, 23: 605.

OSHA. Occupational Safety and Health Administration, 200 Constitution Ave. NW, Room N2439, Washington, D.C. 20402.

Pearce, J.A. Skin pressure distributions on three methods of patient support. In *Air-Fluidized Bed Clinical and Research Symposium.* 1971. Artz, C., Ed. Med. University of South Carolina Press, 85-9.

Pearce, J.A. *Electrosurgery.* 1986. Chapman & Hall, London.

Pegum, J.S. Nickel allergy. *Lancet* 1974, April 13: 674.

Randell-Baker, L. and Roberts, R.B. Hazards of ethylene oxide sterilization. *Anesthesiology* 1969: 349–350.

Richardson, D.R., Caravati, C.M., and Weary, P.E. Allergic contact dermatitis to alcohol swabs. *Cutis* 1969, 5: 1115–1118.

Rothwell, K.G. Iodine toxicity. *Ann. Thoracic Surg.* 1980, 42(4): 481.

Rycroft, R.J.G. Canadian sheet dermatitis. *Br. Med. J.* 1976, November 13: 1175.

Schick, J.F. Burn hazard of isopropyl alcohol in the neonate. *Pediatrics* 1981, 68(4): 587–588.

Scott, E.M. and Gorman, S.P. Glutaraldehyde. In *Disinfection, Sterilization and Preservation.* 4th ed. 1991. Block, SS., Eds. Lea & Febiger, Philadelphia.

Sexton, R.J. and Henson R.V. Experimental ethylene oxide human skin injuries. *Arch. Ind. Hygiene* 1950, 25: 549–564.

Shyu, K., Hwang, J., Lin, S., et al. Prospective study of blood cultures during transesophageal echocardiography. *Am. Heart J.* 1992, 124(6): 1541–1544.

Silver, M.L. Sensitivity to bentonite. EEG. *Clin. Neurophysiol.* 1950, 2: 115.

Strahan, R.W. and Simmons, B. Electronystagmographic electrode skin lesions. *Arch. Otolaryngol.* 1968, 88: 152–155.

Storrs, F.J. Para-choloro-meta-xylenol allergic contact dermatitis in seven individuals. *Contact Dermatitis* 1975, 1: 211–213.

Van Ketel, W.G. and Tan-Lim, K.N. Contact dermatitis from alcohol. *Contact Dermatitis* 1975, 1: 7–10.

Watt, T.L. and Baumann, R.R. Nickel earlobe dermatitis. *Arch. Derm.* 1968, 98: 155–158.

White, C.W. Ethylene oxide sterilization of anesthesia equipment. *Anesthesiology* 1970, 33: 120.

9 Experiences That May Help Technical Experts

CONTENTS

INTRODUCTION

During the last decade and a half, I have served as an expert witness in lawsuits related to patent infringement and invalidation, libel, trade secrets, medical device accidents, and industrial accidents. These cases brought me into contact with a large number of attorneys and quite a few judges. I learned a lot about the legal process and lawyers and hereby share some experiences that may help other technical experts. Most of my experience has been in two areas: (1) medical device accidents and (2) patent infringement and invalidation. After discussing these topics, I will dwell on various items of interest to a technical expert.

MEDICAL DEVICE ACCIDENTS

An accident is defined as an undesirable or unfortunate happening or anything that occurs unexpectedly. Medical devices embrace a very broad range of technologies and therefore accidents occur in many medical specialties, such as surgery, radiology, obstetrics, gynecology, neonatology, cardiology, respiratory therapy, orthopedics, etc. Although most of the accidents associated with these medical specialties occur in the hospital or clinic, out-of-hospital accidents are associated with implanted devices, such as cardiac pacemakers, defibrillators, heart valves, orthopedic implants, silicone implants, etc. It is anticipated that with the increase in home health care, accidents in the home and nursing home will increase. Special knowledge, investigative skills, and tact are required to identify the causes of accidents in these various areas.

ACCIDENT INVESTIGATION

The goal of an accident investigation is to determine what happened, how it happened, and why it happened. The goal is not to establish blame. A secondary goal is to make recommendations so that the risk of a subsequent accident is minimized. The sooner the investigation after the accident, the more likely it is to obtain reliable information; memory dims with the passage of time.

An accident investigation is a search for the truth. There are two aspects to a medical-device accident investigation: (1) examination and testing of the accused device and (2) seeking relevant information about the accident. Soon after the accident, an Incident Report and a Medical Device Report are filed. The accused device and its accessories are impounded and time starts to pass as litigation commences.

It is important to collect critical pieces of information. For example, if the accident site is visited, it is necessary to obtain the address and room number of the organization and the names, occupations, and telephone numbers of those present and interviewed. Sketches of the scene and photographs are very useful in reconstructing the accident. If a piece of equipment is involved, note its type, serial number, and manufacturer. If a piece of equipment is sent to you, write down the date of receipt, the name of the manufacturer, and the model and serial number before examining the device. Then compose a short narrative that describes the state of the device when you received it. Sketches and measurements are useful if there is visible damage. Identify the name and telephone number of the person who sent you the device, the date that it was sent, and the means of conveyance to you. Many useful suggestions on accident investigation are given in a book by Shepherd (1992) and in a chapter by Bruley (1996).

It is always necessary to determine if the accused device malfunctioned, and nondestructive testing is instituted. Obviously, the plaintiff, the defendant(s), and the manufacturer are involved. It is common for the testing to be performed in the presence of representatives (e.g., expert witnesses) for the plaintiff and defendant. Sometimes a third party (e.g., a testing laboratory) is used for the tests. Occasionally, one of the expert witnesses will perform the testing in the presence of the other party. Sometimes the manufacturer is sent the device for testing to determine if it performs according to manufacturer's specifications and existing standards.

Medical device accidents occur long before litigation begins; a delay of 1 to 2 years is not uncommon before the expert witness becomes involved. However, there exist documents that were composed at the time of the accident. For example, it is mandatory that a dated Incident Report and a Medical Device Report (MDR) be completed; both can be made available and contain valuable information relative to an accident. In fact, it is possible to obtain a file of MDRs on the accused device from the FDA. Additional information can be obtained from medical records, including operative, anesthesia, and recovery-room reports when applicable. The patient's admission and discharge record and nurse's progress notes often contain useful information. Depositions taken from those present at the time of the accident are especially useful in putting together the events that led to the accident, as well as providing additional information on the accident.

PATENTS, INFRINGEMENT, AND INVALIDATION

Considerable litigation can be associated with infringement of a patent for a medical device and often technical expert witnesses are hired by both the plaintiff and defendant. The following will address some of the more important issues related to patent infringement and patent invalidation. Briefly, infringement involves making, using, or selling a product covered by claims in an issued patent. Invalidation seeks to show that the art described in the issued patent was known previously and/or obvious to one skilled in the art at that time.

PATENTS

A U.S. patent is a contract between the inventor and the people of the U.S. represented by the U.S. Patent and Trademark Office. The right conferred upon the inventor is the right to exclude others from making, using, or selling that which is covered in the claims of the patent. Such rights are really restricted rights in the sense that the patentee is not given the right to do anything except exclude others from *making*, *using*, or *selling* the invention for a limited time. In exchange for the rights granted by the government, the inventor is required to provide a complete disclosure of the invention. This is the inventor's value surrendered as part of the contractual agreement. Public disclosure of the invention is made when the patent issues.

The general subject matter to which patents are directed is considered to be the useful art. Patents are granted for inventions directed to processes, machines, manufactures, or composition of matter, or any new and useful improvements thereof. Briefly, eligibility for a patent requires that a useful problem is solved, the solution is novel, and the concept is not obvious to one skilled in the art.

An issued patent identifies the inventor(s), cites prior art (patents and/or publications), contains an abstract, figures, specification, and claims. The specification provides a detailed explanation of the invention, including a description of all figures. The specification may include a description of how the invention overcomes problems in the prior art and identifies one or more preferred embodiments of the invention. The claims, which appear at the end of the patent, point out and distinctly assert title to the subject matter that the applicant considers to be his/her contribution or invention for which he/she received the patent. It is the claim or claims that are compared to the prior art to determine patentability. Likewise, it is the claim or claims that are compared to an accused infringement to determine if infringement exists.

Recall that a patent prevents others from making, using, and/or selling something that solves a problem, and that is novel and not obvious to one skilled in the art. The patent claims provide the basis for an infringement lawsuit. It is the way the claims are interpreted in view of the alleged infringement that creates the controversy which is settled by litigation.

The problem solved by the invention is always apparent; however, interpretations of "obvious" and "one skilled in the art" become important issues. Webster's dictionary defines obvious as: (1) open to view or knowledge, and (2) being or standing in the way; the following synonyms are provided: plain, manifest, and evident. One litigious client of mine defined obvious as that which an ordinary person could see and understand.

One skilled in the art is difficult to define. However, a quotation from Jacob Leuopold (1726), translated by Hoff and Geddes (1962), may still be timely. Leuopold stated:

> A mechanic ought to be a person who not only understands well and thoroughly all handicrafts, such as wood, steel, iron, brass, silver, gold, glass, and all such materials to be treated according to the arts, and who knows how to judge on physical principles, how far each according to its nature and property is adequate or suitable to withstand and endure this or that, so that everything receives its necessary proportion, strength, and convenience, and neither too much nor too little is done in the matter; but he must also be able to arrange according to mechanical sciences or rules for any required proportion, or effect according to present or proposed force or load; for which purpose he must also have learned from geometry and arithmetic all that is necessary for calculation of the parts of the machine. And when he desires thoroughly to understand his profession, he must have a complete grasp of all the arts and professions for which he will have to make and invent machines; for otherwise he knows not what he is doing, and has also no power to improve anything, or invent anything new, such as is chiefly demanded of a mechanic. But above all he has to be a born mechanic, so that he shall not only be skilled in invention by natural instinct, but shall also grasp with little trouble all arts and sciences, in such a way that it may be said of him: what his eyes see, that also his hands are able to do; and that love of his art lets him avoid no trouble, labor, or cost, because throughout his whole life he has daily to learn something new and to experiment.

PATENT INFRINGEMENT

It is the obligation of the owner of a patent (or the licensee) to prove that claims or elements in the claims of his/her issued patent are infringed by an accused infringer. The infringed claims are identified by number and the litigation begins. Sometimes the number of infringed claims is reduced as the attorneys communicate. If an accused product fails to include even a single element (or its equivalent) of a claim, there can be no infringement of that claim either literally or under the Doctrine of Equivalents. In other words, the plaintiff must prove that at least one of the cited claims and the elements therein are infringed. Thus, it is interpretation of the claim language that becomes the central focus and the Doctrine of Equivalents is invoked.

Briefly, this doctrine states that infringement exists if the accused infringing production process does substantially the same thing in substantially the same manner and accomplishes substantially the same result as that afforded by the patent claims. Webster's dictionary defines substantial as of a corporeal or material nature, real or actual, of ample or considerable amount, quantity, size, etc. What constitutes equivalence must be determined in the context of the patent, the prior art, and the particular circumstances of the case. An important part of an infringement case is court rulings in prior cases that may take precedent.

Often the issue of interchangeabilty is raised when infringement is being argued. Obviously, if an important component in the alleged infringing device is interchangeable with a component in the invention, it is difficult to argue that there is no infringement. However, if the component in the alleged infringing device, when substituted into the invented device, will not perform and achieve substantially the same result, noninfringement can be argued.

PATENT INVALIDATION

A second line of defense that an alleged patent infringer may take is to show that the issued patent that is allegedly infringed is invalid. Often efforts to prove noninfringement and invalidity progress simultaneously. For the patentee, the possibility of discovering that his/her patent may be invalid is troublesome. Before discussing invalidity, it is appropriate to view the duties of a patent examiner to show what underlies granting a patent.

A patent application receives very close scrutiny by one or more examiners; however, it is only the Primary Examiner who can grant or deny a patent. Patent examiners have special knowledge, training, and skills which are aided by an enormous amount of cross-indexed documents. The U.S. Patent and Trademark Office has access to 30 million documents, more than 5 million U.S. patents, 3 million foreign patents, and a library of 120 million publications. A Primary Examiner will have trained at a Patent Academy and had 7 years of on-the-job training to back up his/her decision to issue or deny a patent. However, before issuing a patent, the examiner has responded to the applicant via documents known as "office action". In the absence of prior art turning up in the search, the Primary Examiner must judge whether the invention is not obvious to one skilled in the art. It is often this situation that is attacked by those seeking to invalidate a patent.

From the foregoing, it is clear that the absence of prior art and nonobviousness to one skilled in the art, in full view of the prior art, are what make an invention patentable. Thus, invalidation must address these issues and the burden of proof of invalidation lies with the alleged infringer.

If an inventor, either willfully or negligently, fails to disclose material prior art to the examiner, a case for invalidation can be made, particularly if it can be shown that the inventor possessed such information. I remember one case in which an inventor desired to obtain FDA approval for the sale of a medical device and avoid lengthy clinical testing by stating in the FDA application that the inventor's device was substantially the same as an FDA-approved device. The interesting fact is that the FDA-approved device was in use before the inventor filed for a patent.

Other ways of showing that an inventor may have concealed important background information is to read his/her publications and those cited in the patent. In addition, it is useful to read the papers that appear in the references of the papers identified in the patent. Bibliographic thoroughness requires that all relevant references must have been read and understood.

Dealing with the issue of "obvious to one skilled in the art" is more difficult and requires knowledge of the state of the art when the inventor applied for the patent. It also requires a knowledge of how others solved the same problem as claimed in the invention. Although there are other legal issues associated with invalidation, in the final analysis, interpretation of the submitted evidence is subjective; therefore, it is necessary to produce evidence that is easily understood by a judge and jury. This is especially important because every patent comes a presumption of validity that can only be overcome by clear and convincing evidence.

THE TECHNICAL EXPERT

A technical expert can be used in two ways: (1) as a fact witness and (2) as an expert witness. In the former case, the expert provides facts, not opinions. Facts are derived from published papers, books, patents, documents, etc. along with perhaps a summary of existing knowledge that is accepted by those in the field. On the other hand, the expert witness does the same and, using this information, provides an opinion based on facts, training, and experience. Interestingly enough, in the courtroom, it is only the expert witness and the jury who are entitled to provide an opinion. The judge acts as a chairperson who guides the proceedings that lead to exposition of the truth. In those cases where there is no jury, the judge can render an opinion based on the facts established by the attorneys for the plaintiff and the defense.

The single most important talent that an expert witness must have is the ability to teach technical material to nontechnical people, namely, the judge and jury. Prior to this activity he/she has been teaching the attorney who hired the expert. The better informed the attorney, the better he/she is able to frame questions to achieve delivery of the facts, know what to emphasize, and know how to shoot down opponents who attempt to bring in confusing, misleading, or irrelevant material. There is no substitute for a good rapport with the attorney who engaged your services.

The first fact to be ascertained is whether you are serving on behalf of the plaintiff or defendant. Sometimes, in the very early stage of a lawsuit, this information may not come automatically. On some occasions an attorney will telephone and describe the case briefly and inquire about the documents that you would like to examine. When they arrive, it is clear for which side you are serving. It is important to discover which points your attorney wishes to establish so that you can focus your attention on documents that support the attorney's viewpoint. Sometimes contrary information is adduced and this, too, must be communicated to your attorney. Usually additional documents are needed to establish the cause of an accident and the technical expert requests that the attorney obtain them.

In cases where there are multiple defendants, it is sometimes unclear (at least in the beginning) which defendant is most vulnerable. Although several experts may be on the side where there are multiple defendants, an expert serves for only the hiring attorney. I have never experienced multiple attorneys on the same side pooling their expert witness resources.

ATTORNEYS

It is useful to recognize that there are two types of attorney: (1) those who want the truth even if it is injurious to his/her case, and (2) those who want the expert to say whatever is necessary to win the case. The former type wants no surprise during the lawsuit or in court; the latter runs the risk of damage to the case during deposition or during cross-examination in the courtroom. The prudent expert knows that the truth, and documented evidence, are essential and unassailable.

DISCOVERY

During discovery, the pretrial time, both sides are pressed to acquire pertinent information. During this time it is unwise to write anything down that could reveal your opinion. What I have found to be very useful is to compose a table of contents for each document that I have read and staple this table to the document. In this way, I can gain easy access (by page number) to any fact or statement made that is pertinent to the case. When evidence is contained in scientific papers, I index each in the same way to identify where the useful information is to be found. The availability of such inventories makes it easy to refresh one's memory and prepare for deposition and the courtroom.

THE REPORT

Rule 26 of the Federal Rules of Civil Procedure gives a detailed account the requirements for the report of an expert witness and this document should be consulted. The essence of this rule is as follows:

> The report shall contain a complete statement of all opinions to be expressed and the basis and reasons therefore; the data or other information considered by the witness in forming the opinions; any exhibits to be used as a summary of or support for the opinions; the qualifications of the witness, including a list of all publications authored by the witness within the preceding ten years; the compensation to be paid for the study and testimony; and a listing of any other cases in which the witness has testified as an expert at trial or by deposition within the preceding four years.

Although Rule 26 requires provision of considerable information, much of it will have been requested by the hiring attorney long before a final written report is requested.

Often during pursuit of a case, a report is often requested by the attorney that you serve. While it is true that attorneys use the same English language as we mortals, they use it differently and punctuate long sentences differently. Therefore, the report has to be in the form that is unambiguous to the opposing lawyer. Whereas, when the expert collects and interprets the facts, it requires a collaborative effort between an expert witness and an attorney to get the report in a form and style understandable to all attorneys. For example, suppose that X was the critical item that caused injury. An attorney would state that the accused did not know X and should have, or if the accused knew X, it was disregarded and it was this disregard that caused the accident that caused the injury. From the foregoing, the expert witness must recognize that his/her facts and evidence must be assembled and presented in a style that is very different from that used in scientific reports and publications. I have found that the best way to start a report is by a telephone conversation with the attorney that you serve. Then a rough draft is composed by you and either read to the attorney or sent to him/her by FAX. This iterative process may continue four or five times before the final report is created. Meeting with your attorney in person to collaborate on the report is very desirable, but this is rarely possible. Remember that this report is made available to opposing counsel. Unlike Perry Mason trials in which a new piece of evidence appears first in court, in the real world, both sides work from the same body of evidence; what makes it interesting is to see how different interpretations are placed on the same evidence. Be aware that your report is a statement of your opinion and, along with any deposition, it will be used in the courtroom. As a result of the Daubert vs. Merrell Dow case in 1993, scientific evidence is required to support your expert opinion. For example, the expert's opinion must be supported by scientific reasoning and methodology that is generally accepted in the expert's particular scientific community. Obviously, the scientific data must be reliable. Stated differently, general scientific knowledge and published literature are needed to justify, to a reasonable certainty, your expert opinion. Obviously, it is necessary to show that the cited scientific knowledge and published literature apply directly to this case.

Although there is no standard form for the final report, it must contain certain key pieces of information. Most importantly, the report must inventory all case documents examined by you. The final report must provide a summary of the basis for the lawsuit, i.e., a description of the accident, the basis for a patent infringement, etc. Finally, the report states your opinion and the basis for it. The following fictitious example is presented for guidance.

Date

Robert L. Brown
Rouge, Weiss & Azul
0001 Highwater Street
Schwartbert NWT
H270-A66-WL20

RE: Blanco vs. Knife & Omnihospital

Dear Mr. Brown,

I have examined the following documents that pertain to this case:

1. Surgeon Knife's report
2. Operating Room record
3. Anesthesia record
4. Incident Report
5. Deposition of Dr. Right
6. Deposition by Dr. Fence
7. Medical records of Blanco

Brief Description:

On 9/31/92, Jason Blanco, a 30-year-old male, underwent endoscopic surgery to remove his gallbladder. The operation was performed under general anesthesia by Dr. Knife, a staff surgeon at the Omnihospital. Electrosurgery was used to cut and coagulate and the dispersive electrode was on the anterior right thigh. A standard model X225P dispersive electrode was used which has been used by this hospital for the last 5 years. During the surgery, Knife noted that at the start of the operation, cutting and coagulation were satisfactory; but later, cutting and coagulation were both a little "slow". Therefore, the surgeon requested more output from the electro-surgical unit. The operation progressed without incident and was completed success-fully in 2.5 h. However, when the drapes and the electrosurgical electrode were removed, it was noted that there was a 3×3-cm burn on the right thigh, characterized by second- and third-degree (full-thickness) burns. On consultation with the family, debridement and skin grafting were decided upon and performed successfully the next day by Dr. Right.

Analysis: The function of an electrosurgical dispersive electrode (Bovie pad) is to provide a safe return path for the electrosurgical current to the electrosurgical unit (ESU). It does so by providing a large area of contact with the skin. A typical dispersive electrode is 4×6 in. (10×15 cm). There is an AAMI/ANSI standard of performance for such electrodes and all that are available commercially must meet this standard. If the skin contact area is reduced, all of the current is forced to pass through a smaller area (current crowding); the current density (mA/cm^2) will be high and skin heating will occur. The amount of heating depends on the current density (squared), the intensity of the electrosurgical current, and how long it flows, which depends on the number of activations of the ESU.

In relating these facts to the Blanco incident, note that the burn measured 3×3 cm, which is much smaller than the size of a typical electrosurgical electrode (10×15 cm); therefore, the area of skin contact was small, favoring heat production. If we use the burn area ($3 \times 3 = 9$ cm^2) as the effective contact area, this area is only 6% of the area of a typical dispersive electrode (150 cm^2).

In addition, during the operation, the surgeon requested more output from the ESU. This is consistent with the development of a small area of contact which would increase the resistance and require a higher output setting on the ESU, which was requested by Dr. Knife.

Dr. Fence, expert for the defendant, argues that the electrode was defective, but provides no proof. The fact that the hospital has been using the same type of electrode for the last 5 years without incident argues against a defective electrode design. Also, the fact that cutting and coagulation difficulties were not present earlier in the procedure argues against a defective electrode and points to partial dislodgment of the electrode during the operation.

In summary, the electrode contact area with Blanco's skin was small, which caused current crowding, and it was the current crowding that produced the heating that produced the second- and third-degree burns. When a surgeon encounters poor cutting and coagulating, good practice requires that the dispersive electrode and all cables to the ESU and the ESU be checked before proceeding.

Respectfully submitted,

Pietro Amaretto, PhD, PE, etc.
State License Number
Social Security Number

In a report or an affidavit, it is useful to keep the door open to accommodate new, unanticipated, admissible evidence that may come in the future. Therefore, it may be of value to consider inclusion of the following sentence: "I reserve the right to modify or change the opinions and conclusions upon the discovery of additional information, facts, and other circumstances discovered during dependency of any litigation relating to this matter."

Attorneys rely heavily on precedents and I have found that it is often possible to bring a case to a climax without the need of a report by scouring the published literature to find prior publications that deal directly with the events in the present case. For example, I have found papers that describe a medical device accident that is the same as the one being litigated. I have also found publications that reveal prior art that bears directly on patent invalidation. However, it is not enough to find such publications; it is necessary to identify in them the relevant paragraphs or statements. Attorneys take such material seriously and its presentation has often resulted in prompt settlement.

THE DEPOSITION

The deposition of an expert is an interrogation taken under oath by the opposing attorney. All questions and answers are recorded by a court reporter. Prior to the deposition, make a list of all documents that you have examined that pertain to the case because you will be asked for this information. Just before the deposition begins, take a few minutes with the court reporter to identify technical terms and their spelling, as well as abbreviations and acronyms. This investment in time will pay off later when you proofread your sworn deposition.

The attorney who hired you is present at the deposition. The objective of the opposing attorney is to discover your opinion, which you guard carefully. In other words, the opposing attorney wants to know what you think by asking artfully composed questions which are answered truthfully without commentary; give nothing away. You have no obligation to educate the opposing attorney. If his/her questions are unclear or misleading, ask for a repetition or a rephrasing. Although your attorney will object to some questions, these objections are usually only for the record. Occasionally, some questions violate the rules of procedure and are objected to strenuously. Try to avoid giving a strong conclusion at this time because you may be dealing with limited data. By trial time, new admissible information may be adduced which may or may not modify your opinion. Also recognize that some new evidence may not be admissible. Proofread the typed deposition and remember that the opposing attorney can use this document in court; therefore, you must be consistent. During cross-examination, never guess or speculate; merely state, "I do not remember" or "I do not know."

Sworn depositions can be taken anywhere. Typically, they are taken in the offices of the attorney for the defense or plaintiff. Sometimes a deposition is videotaped. I have been deposed in a meeting room in an out-of-town hotel agreed upon by the attorneys. I have had my deposition taken via a conference telephone call. In such a case, the attorney that I serve was with me and all relevant documents and exhibits were present at both sites. This method is very convenient and quite inexpensive, in view of the high cost of air travel and time loss due to travel.

CHRONOLOGY OF A CASE

Lawsuits do not progress swiftly, nor do all cases go to trial. It is reliably estimated that more than 95% of all lawsuits are settled out of court. However, it is rarely possible to predict those that will proceed to trial. Even if a trial date is set, it may be delayed for weeks or months. Even if the trial date is changed several times, it is still not possible to predict that a trial will be held. I have experienced settlement of a lawsuit before testifying on the first day of trial. Nonetheless, if a trial date is set, be fully prepared to testify in the courtroom then.

The time course of a lawsuit often shares what I call the airport syndrome "hurry up and wait." Typically, an attorney has about one half dozen active cases — all with differing urgencies. Witnesses have to be interrogated, documents have to be located and analyzed, depositions have to be taken, and court hearings have to be scheduled. A technical expert may enter early or late in these proceedings and often is asked for a prompt preliminary opinion. Frequently, the expert hears nothing and wonders what, if anything, is going on. A phone call to the attorney will solve this problem and may reveal that you need to be in court in 3 weeks, or, as is more usual, the trial has been set for a date that is about 10 months in the future. I have one case that is 2 years old and another that is more than 4 years old; with both it is impossible to estimate a trial date. Such a situation is usually frustrating to a technical expert who is used to solving problems with dispatch. However, take it easy on your ulcers and blood pressure. Develop a tolerant attitude because the process is not likely to change soon — nor can you change it!

THE COURTROOM

Despite the fact that the witness box is a stressful site for the expert witness, the courtroom is an exciting place where the truth is sought. An enormous amount of information is produced by the attorneys for the plaintiff and defense. There is a considerable amount of information in the behavior of the participants (judge, jury, attorneys, and witnesses). Body language abounds and communicates much information to the sensitive observer. There is considerable information in the time taken to respond to questions as well as how the response is delivered. As is well known, many attorneys can conduct themselves in a threatening or conciliatory manner, depending on what suits them. It can be said that courtroom proceedings can be characterized as a shower of information.

In the courtroom, the role of the expert witness is that of a teacher who is relaxed and has obvious enthusiasm for his/her specialty. Judges and jurors are nontechnical people, by and large, and it is the duty of the expert to translate technical material into simple and easy-to-understand concepts. I have found that charts, large illustrations, models, videotapes, and demonstrations in the courtroom are very effective. However, never schedule a demonstration if there is even the slightest chance of failure — make a videotape of the demonstration under conditions that you control.

When interrogated, be relaxed; present your answers to the jury, not the attorney. Engage the jury with eye contact and maintain their attention. Be animated, enthusiastic, and show that you are happy to be there to reveal the truth. The first few minutes of direct examination are the most important because your attorney is guiding you with his questions and these are designed to make your points. This is your chance to tell your story. A good attorney will not ask you a leading question, which is one that contains the answer. This is called "leading the witness" and will be objected to. The cross-examiner will try to discredit you, confuse you, and show that you are inconsistent in every way that he/she can. Be sure of your facts and beliefs, hold your ground, and the cross-examiner cannot win.

In the courtroom one encounters many different interrogation styles. For example, there is Loudmouth who shouts his/her questions at you, which is a tactic designed to rattle or intimidate you. The best defense is to give your answer in a soft, confident voice; this will expose Loudmouth's strategy. Give your answer by directing your attention to the jury or judge, not to Loudmouth.

Binary is the type of attorney who demands a yes-or-no answer to each question. Binary uses this technique to filter the information that you can provide. Binary often interrupts your answers, demanding the yes-or-no answer. The best way of dealing with Binary is to look at the judge or jury and say, "A yes-or-no answer will not reveal the truth."

The Assumer is an attorney who directs the expert to assume something that is very likely contrary to his/her opinion. Beware of the Assumer; he/she will build on the assumption and coax you to agree. On occasion I have refused to join in the assumption, stating that it is too hypothetical or speculative. Only on one occasion has the judge requested me to assume. I balked stating that the assumption would go contrary to my belief.

The Fisherman, who is looking for information, is an attorney who asks questions that are barely relevant and usually call for an affirmative response. The questions often deal with what a prudent person would do or think. By this strategy the Fisherman is trying to cloud the issue by showing how often you agree. A jury could begin to think that you are inconsistent or agree, in general, with Fisherman. You must make your answers bring the questioning back to the central issue — or show tactfully that the central issue is not being addressed.

Double Negative is an attorney who uses two negatives in each question. For example, "Do you not think that X would not do that?" Because such questions are confusing to the jury and may even cause the expert to unknowingly misunderstand and/or slip, I have flatly refused to answer such questions and request rephrasing the question without negatives; I have always been accommodated.

Beware of the Machine Gun attorney who is one who repeats the same question many times in rapid fire. He/she knows something that will reveal that you are inconsistent. A typical question is, "You never said (or did) X?" He/she knows you did and is waiting for you to say that you never said (or did) X. The best answer is "I don't recall."

You, as an expert witness, are at the mercy of the cross-examiner. However, you are not entirely defenseless. Having the truth on your side is the best defense. You can easily rattle the cross-examiner by stating, when appropriate, "That is an excellent question, I am glad that you asked it." Believe me, the cross-examiner will change the subject quickly to prevent you from making points with the judge and jury.

Jury trials are held in the courtroom in the presence of the judge, jury, and attorneys for the plaintiff and defense. Expert witnesses are usually excluded until they are called upon to testify. However, not all such trials have all of the parties in the courtroom. One trial in which I participated employed two-way videoconference equipment. I, the expert witness, and my attorney were in a city 1000 mi from the courtroom. I could see the judge and attorneys in the courtroom and those in the courtroom could see me. There was no jury on this case. Two-way audio and graphics display capability completed the facilities. The graphics display allowed large-screen showing of exhibits and documents.

Two-way videoconference is now not expensive when compared to the cost of air travel and hotel expenses. A video technician is required at each end of the circuit and, in addition to their hourly cost, there is an equipment setup and rental charge, plus an hourly rate for the two-way communication circuit.

Whether two-way videoconference facilities will be allowed is up to the judge. First, the plaintiff and defense attorneys must agree; then they petition the judge. In the case just referred to, I was a scheduled expert witness with an illness that prevented me from traveling to the courtroom.

PAYMENT FOR SERVICES

As stated previously, lawsuits do not proceed with the speed of sound. In accident cases I am called as an expert witness, typically 2 years after the incident. I have had similar experiences with patent-infringement and libel cases. During this time attorneys for both sides have been accumulating information and documents. A point is reached when an attorney wants an expert to evaluate the information, often as quickly as possible via a telephone conversation. At this point it is prudent to describe your evaluation as preliminary because more information is likely to appear as witnesses are deposed. Thus starts an ongoing process in which the expert starts to devote time periodically to the case; this makes it necessary to establish a schedule for billing. Many experts bill on a monthly basis; but this is not always practical because a lawsuit does not proceed at a uniform rate.

Colleagues of mine have reported to me a situation which is troublesome that relates to billing. Typically, at the outset, an attorney will inquire about your hourly charges and request a curriculum vitae and list of publications. It is important to identify those publications that pertain to the case at hand. Also important is identification of experience that you have had in the area of the present case. By providing this information, the attorney can identify your value to the case at hand.

I have been told that some attorneys use your curriculum vitae and publication list to arrange a settlement and often do not report back to the expert. As a result, some expert witnesses charge for sending their curriculum vitae and list of publications. Fortunately, I have not had such an experience.

The trial is over or a summary judgment has occurred, or the parties have had a settlement conference and the lawsuit is ended. Now you need to be paid. Perhaps you have had an advance, perhaps you have billed periodically during the litigation, or perhaps you elected to wait until the suit is over; this latter is not to be recommended. The following paragraphs refer to the financial aspects of the activities of an expert witness.

Regarding remuneration for services rendered, there is no standard method. Some attorneys provide an advance as a retainer, usually $500 to $1000. Because lawsuits may carry on for years, it is wise to submit an invoice periodically. It is often easy to identify when critical phases have passed. I usually submit an invoice after each phase. The invoice identifies the litigants, the time covered by the services, and any expenses incurred. The invoice includes my name, degrees, social security number, and license numbers.

In providing payment, there are two types of procedure. With one, the attorney or his/her law firm issues a check on its account. With the other, the attorney sends the invoice to the organization that hired the law firm. This procedure delays payment considerably. In one case that I had, it took 6 months to be paid. To keep the issue alive, I submitted (to the law firm) an invoice each month, marking them second notice (with date), third notice (with date), etc. The final (sixth) invoice carried the dates of all six invoices and was such an embarrassment that payment was received and the second notice was attached to the check! The message here is "erosion will ultimately win."

Sometimes an attorney neglects to respond to your invoices and a phone call will discover the reason. In problem cases you may suggest an installment plan for payment. Somewhat less attractive is to request payment for a reduced amount within 7 days. You may elect to settle via the Small Claims Court. Finally, you may consider filing a complaint with the State Bar Association, claiming nonprofessional conduct.

In 1996 the National Academy of Forensic Engineers (NAFE) published a very useful handbook entitled Business and Financial Practices for Forensic Engineers. In it are chapters on the code of ethics for forensic engineers, risk management, insurance for errors and omissions (E and O), record keeping, financial management, fees and collection thereof, and marketing your services. This 102-page book contains a wealth of information derived from the practice of forensic engineering.

WHERE TO FIND INFORMATION

MEDICAL DEVICE ACCIDENTS

Attorneys and expert witnesses always want to know if the accident under investigation is common or rare, or if there are precedents that could effect a judgment. Such background information is not always easy to locate. There are many sources of information on medical device accidents. As stated earlier, Medical Device Reports (MDRs), which describe an accident, are available from the Food and Drug Administration (FDA). Institutional medical records, the Incident Report, and depositions obtained from those present at the time of the accident contain valuable information. A book by Gendron (1988) contains descriptions of a large number of different types of accidents and includes references to original sources. In some cases, the court rulings are provided. The book by Shepherd (1992) also contains accident descriptions and identifies the types of questions that should be asked to investigate the accident to determine the cause. A monograph by Geddes (1995), which deals with the response of living tissue to the passage of direct current and low- and high-frequency alternating current, also contains descriptions of medical device accidents due to such currents. The Emergency Care Research Institute (ECRI) maintains a very large data base on medical accidents. ECRI also publishes a journal entitled *Health Devices* that contains accident reports.

Information on accidents related to anesthesia is available from the American Society of Anesthesiologists, which maintains a Closed Claims Data Base. A wide variety of accidents that occurred during anesthesia are described therein. In addition, the Wood Library — Museum of Anesthesiology also maintains a data base of anesthesia accidents.

Published papers on accidents can be accessed through a library search of key words. Although the practice of listing key words is of more recent origin, the references in the recent publications provide the trail to previous accidents of the same type.

MEDICAL DEVICE STANDARDS

Before the FDA was given authority to regulate medical devices in 1976, the various professional societies had made recommendations for minimum performance of devices. In parallel with these activities, several industrial standards-promulgating groups, notably, the National Fire Protection Association and the Underwriters Laboratory, concerned themselves with the safety of medical devices. Now there are mandatory standards for efficacy and safety for medical devices which resulted from the activities of the FDA Device Classification Panels. The Association for the Advancement of Medical Instrumentation (AAMI) in collaboration with the American National Standards Institute (ANSI) maintains a file of the latest AAMI/ANSI standards for the safety and efficacy of medical devices. The American Society for Testing Materials (ASTM) has promulgated performance standards for certain medical devices. The Electronic Industries Association (EIA) concerns itself with the safety of medical devices. There are many professional organizations in the U.S. that concern themselves with promoting safe medical equipment. The analog of the FDA in Canada is the Canadian Standards Association (CSA) and in Europe, the International Electrotechnical Commission (IEC); both promulgate medical device standards. The IEC has a wider range of performance standards than is required in the U.S., and when a U.S. standard is absent, the IEC standard is often cited. In addition to AAMI, ANSI, and ASTM, a wide variety of standards documents can be obtained from Global Engineering Documents.

LEGAL DOCUMENTS

There are two enormous data bases that cover the legal aspects of medical mishaps, as well as a wide variety of other subjects, including patents and patent infringement cases. The Lexis-Nexis data base serves 60 countries and has 7300 data bases and adds 9.5 million documents each week. Both legal and nonlegal information is available. The West Publishing Co. operates the WestDoc data base and contains federal and state case law entries. Attorney editorial services can be provided and a nominal charge is levied for each case, there being no subscription fees. Lexis-Nexis and West Doc are the data bases that attorneys search.

REFERENCES

AAMI — Association for the Advancement of Medical Instrumentation. 3330 Washington Blvd., Arlington, VA 22201-4598.
American Society of Anesthesiologists. 520 N. Northwest Highway, Park Ridge, IL 60068-2573, <http: //ASAhq.org>.
American National Standards Institute. 1430 Broadway, New York.
Bruley, M.E. Accident and forensic investigation. In *Medical Devices*. 1966. Van Gruting, C.W.D., Ed. Elsevier Science BV, Amsterdam, The Netherlands.
Canadian Standards Association. 235 Montreal Rd., Ottawa, Canada K1A 0L2.
Electronic Industries Association (EIA), Health Care Electronics Section. 2001 Eye Street, N.W., Washington, D.C. 20006.
Emergency Care Research Institute (ECRI). 5200 Butler Pike, Plymouth Meeting, PA 19462.
Food and Drug Administration. 5600 Fisher's Lane, Rockville, MD 20857.
Geddes, L.A. *Handbook of Electrical Hazards and Accidents*. 1995. CRC Press, Boca Raton, FL.
Gendron, F.C. *Unexplained Patient Burns*. 1988. Quest Publishing (now Lippincott-Raven Press), Brea, CA.
Global Engineering Documents. Clayton, MO.
Hoff, H.E. and Geddes, L.A. The beginnings of graphic recording. *ISIS* 1962, 53, Part 3(173): 287–324.
International Electrotechnical Commission (IEC). Centre du Service Clientele (CSC), Commission Electrotechnique Internationale, 3, rue do Varembe, Case postale 131, CH1211-Geneve 20 (Geneva) Suisse (Switzerland).
Lexis-Nexis. 9443 Springboro Pike, PO Box 933, Dayton, OH 45401.
National Academy of Forensic Engineers. 174 Brady Avenue, Hawthorne, NY 10532.
National Fire Protection Association. 470 Atlantic Ave, Boston, MA 02210.

Shepherd, M.D. *Shepherd's System for Medical Device Investigation and Reporting.* 1992. Quest Publishing (now Lippincott-Raven Press), Brea, CA.

West Publishing Company. 620 Opperman Drive, PO Box 64779, St. Paul, MN 55164-0779, webmaster.westdoc@westpub.com.

Wood Library — Museum of Anesthesiology, 520 Northwest Highway, Park Ridge, 60068-2573, ASA Web page, http: //ASAhq.org and e-mail to: WLM @ASAhq.org. geddes.pap.techexp.5/27.

Index

A